Cerebral Palsy

MANAGEMENT OF DISABILITY
Series editors: Margaret Edwards, Jean Cooper and Robert Ringel

This is the first volume in a new series dealing with the management of various disabilities. The emphasis throughout will be on a team approach and the books will all be written by various members of the team.

Titles in this series

Cerebral Palsy
The child and young person
Edited by L. Cogher, E. Savage and M. F. Smith

Cerebral Palsy
The child and young person

Edited by

Lesley Cogher
Chief Communication Therapist
Elizabeth Savage
Principal Clinical Psychologist
and
Michael F. Smith
Consultant Paediatrician

The Ryegate Children's Centre
Sheffield

CHAPMAN & HALL MEDICAL
London · New York · Tokyo · Melbourne · Madras

Published by Chapman & Hall, 2–6 Boundary Row, London SE1 8HN

Chapman & Hall, 2–6 Boundary Row, London SE1 8HN, UK

Blackie Academic & Professional, Wester Cleddens Road, Bishopbriggs, Glasgow G64 2NZ, UK

Van Nostrand Reinhold Inc., 115 5th Avenue, New York NY10003, USA

Chapman & Hall Japan, Thomson Publishing Japan, Hirakawacho Nemoto Building, 6F, 1-7-11 Hirakawa-cho, Chiyoda-ku, Tokyo 102, Japan

Chapman & Hall Australia, Thomas Nelson Australia, 102 Dodds Street, South Melbourne, Victoria 3205, Australia

Chapman & Hall India, R. Seshadri, 32 Second Main Road, CIT East, Madras 600 035, India

First edition 1992

© 1992 L. Cogher, E. Savage and M. F. Smith

Typeset in 10/12pt Palatino by Best-set Typesetter Ltd., Hong Kong
Printed in Great Britain at the University Press, Cambridge

ISBN 0 412 30900 9

A catalogue record for this book is available from the British Library

Library of Congress Cataloging-in-Publication data available

Contents

Acknowledgements

Major contributions were received from

Dr M. F. Smith, Consultant Paediatrician*
Miss L. Cogher, Chief Communication Therapist*
Miss L. Savage, Principal Clinical Psychologist*
Dr Ruth Powell, Consultant Paediatrician†
Mrs Beryl Seaman, Senior Social Worker‡
Mrs Julie Clarke, Senior Physiotherapist*
Mrs Alison Brown, Senior Occupational Therapist*
Miss Margaret Goodyear, Senior Social Worker*
Mrs Julia Barker, Senior Social Worker*
Mrs Ruth Rudston, Senior Social Worker*
Miss Judith Farren, Head Occupational Therapist*
Mrs May McWilliams, Co-ordinator§
Mr Michael Bell, Consultant Orthopaedic Surgeon‡

Useful contributions were also received from

Miss Doreen Atkinson, Nursing Sister*
Mrs Susan Brett, Senior Physiotherapist*
Mrs Julie Lyons, Senior Physiotherapist*
Miss Angela Churchill, Senior Occupational Therapist*
Mrs Avril Bingley, Support Teacher§
Miss Margaret Sharpe, Support Teacher§
Miss Susie Mitchell, Support Teacher§
Dr Gwilym P. Hosking, Consultant Paediatric Neurologist*
Miss Sue Crane, Senior Speech Therapist*
Mrs Susan Mawson, Senior Physiotherapist‡
Mrs Nicole Sedgwick, Senior Communication Therapist*

*The Ryegate Children's Centre, Sheffield
†Community Child Health, Sheffield Health Anthority
‡The Children's Hospital, Sheffield
§Under 5's Special Needs Service, Sheffield

The authors are indebted to Mrs Pat Winstanley for typing the manuscript and for giving us secretarial support. Pat Bashton, Jackie Buckley, Jayne Flower, Jennie McHale, Jayne Caponcello and Fiona Simpson must also be mentioned for their typing contribution to the earlier stages of the manuscript.

Thanks also to David Forsdike, Rob Quayle and Lynn Rollin for their help and advice in reading and assembling the text.

Preface

In writing this book we have attempted to describe the issues surrounding the diagnosis, assessment, treatment and management of cerebral palsy. Compiled from contributions from the staff of The Ryegate Children's Centre and The Sheffield Children's Hospital, the book reflects not only individual professional knowledge but also experience of working as a team with children with cerebral palsy and their parents. In attempting to present an integrated account of the impact of cerebral palsy on the child and the family's life, it has sometimes been necessary to discuss separate areas of development, but it is hoped that the desirability of a multidisciplinary approach to assessment and remediation is evident.

The book is divided into three parts. The first part attempts to answer the question 'What is cerebral palsy?', to clarify terminology and provide a description of the causes and incidence of the condition.

The second, and major part, is concerned with the impact of cerebral palsy against the background of the developing child and of the challenges faced by all children and their families in the transitions from babyhood to adulthood. We have attempted to present current theoretical perspectives and practical approaches to management, together with insights into the experience of cerebral palsy from the viewpoint of the child and family. The emphasis in this section is on therapeutic and educational strategies which will enable the child to function competently and independently within the family, school and community.

The third and final part deals in more depth with specific issues of assessment and treatment, and includes the assessment of sensory, motor and cognitive functioning together with treatment of epilepsy and surgical intervention. This part is largely based on the approaches used by the team at The Ryegate Children's Centre but also includes a discussion of other philosophies and approaches, and refers the reader to more detailed texts.

The book is intended to be accessible and useful to a wide readership which we hope will include parents of children with cerebral palsy as well as professionals from health, education and social services, who are working with these children. No volume dealing with a condition which has such an extensive and far reaching impact on the child and family can claim to be exhaustive but it is hoped that the broad view taken in this volume will provoke thought and stimulate further reading into the subject.

PART ONE
Classification, Prevalence and Aetiology

1 Classification, prevalence and aetiology

1.1 Definition

Cerebral palsy refers to a group of conditions which share the features of a central motor deficit which is non-progressive pathologically, and which is acquired in early life. Any definition of cerebral palsy encompasses a wide variety of disorders with quite different aetiological and clinical features. This variation occurs across the whole spectrum of cerebral palsy and also within each clinical subgroup.

A problem frequently encountered in definition is the meaning of 'early life'. In surveys of cerebral palsy, there is no consistency as to the inclusion of cases where the disorder is acquired after the neonatal period. In terms of clinical and educational management, this distinction is largely irrelevant. In terms of research into causation and epidemiology, it becomes very important.

A second point concerns the non-progression of the motor deficit. The clinical syndrome of cerebral palsy changes in an individual, with the occurrence of maturation, development and possibly repair. The definition implicitly excludes progressive central nervous system disorders such as tumours and degenerative processes. This changing clinical picture with time is seen, for example, in the child with spastic diplegia, who may initially show poverty of lower limb movement without tonal or reflex changes; there may then be a stage of dystonic posturing with increased reflexes, before the final development of spasticity/rigidity and postural abnormalities. A progression of clinical signs with development is seen in all types of cerebral palsy.

Development, maturation and repair have unpredictable effects in individual children, so that early diagnosis of cerebral palsy may need to be revised as the child matures. For example, with infants thought to be at risk of cerebral palsy (e.g. prematurity, intraventricular haemorrhage), the early identification of abnormal neurological signs may be seen to co-exist with delays in the acquisition of certain motor skills. (This may imply the presence of cerebral palsy.) There is an association of abnormal signs with functional impairment (i.e. delay). In some cases, functional recovery occurs so that, by the second or third year,

Table 1.1   Children who outgrew cerebral palsy (CP)

Diagnosis at 1 year Definite CP		Diagnosis at 7 years		
		No CP	Suspect	Definite
Mild	125	89	4	32
Moderate	71	28	3	40
Severe	33	1	0	32
	229	118	7	104

From Nelson and Ellenberg, 1982.

little or no functional disability can be detected. Abnormal neurological signs may diminish in these children also. In more severely affected children, a diagnosis of cerebral palsy can be achieved in the early months, whereas in less severely affected children caution in diagnosis must be exercised. It is important to observe the progress of the child over some months, very often into the second and occasionally the third year of life, before being sure of a permanent motor deficit. In their large prospective study of neurological signs in children, Nelson and Ellenberg (1982) described the outcome for 37 282 children examined at 1 year and 7 years of age. This important study illustrates that, of 229 children who were thought to have definite cerebral palsy at 1 year of age, 118 (51%) showed a remission of clinical signs by 7 years of age. These authors reported a high incidence of learning difficulties among the cases that remitted, indicating that the earlier abnormal signs reflected cerebral pathology, but that the manifestation of that pathology changed with maturation.

1.2   Classification

Since the early reports by Little (1862), many authorities have attempted to classify the types of cerebral palsy (Ingram, 1964). Proposals have included classification on the basis of:

1. Neuropathological findings at autopsy.
2. Presumed aetiological factors.
3. The clinical neurological syndromes.

Clinicians in practice now classify the cerebral palsies on the basis of the clinical neurological syndromes. The clinical syndromes of cerebral palsy are highly complex and difficult to characterize. There will not be much discussion about diagnosis of hemiplegia, but in cases of

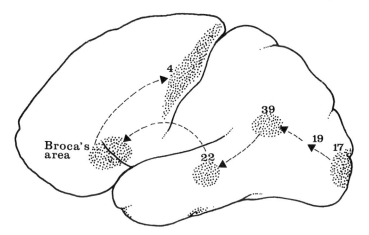

Fig. 1.1 Seeing an object and saying its name (Shepherd, 1988).

diplegia, quadriplegia and dyskinesia, opinions of different examiners frequently vary. The examination of the child will yield a variety of signs, but the frame of reference into which the signs are placed is very variable. So too are the children in terms of their physical signs varying day by day, or even on occasions, hour by hour. In considering the complexity of the motor hierarchy and its disorders, a useful example is that described by Shepherd (1988) – 'seeing an object and saying its name' (Fig. 1.1). This example illustrates the degree of concord in many areas of brain function necessary to perform a particular motor act, in this case naming the object. In this process, visual information from the optic nerves is first received in area 17 of the visual cortex; it is elaborated in area 18 and 19; from there the information is passed to the posterior speech area (Wernicke) of the parietal lobe; from there the information is relayed to the auditory reception area, 22, of the temporal lobe and from there to the anterior speech area of the frontal lobe (Broca's area). From Broca's area, the motor programmes for speech are relayed to the motor cortex. Thus, in order to perform a motor task, a complex series of perceptual manoeuvres needs to be undertaken. The pyramidal and extrapyramidal systems in one sense are merely relay stations in a much more complex motor system: it is not surprising, therefore, that children who have focal or multifocal brain lesions display great variations in physical performance, although the lesions may be superficially similar in different children.

While classification on the basis of the clinical syndrome remains the most useful in the clinical setting, there are two further serious draw-

Table 1.2   Classification of cerebral palsy

Spastic hemiplegia
Spastic diplegia and ataxic diplegia
Spastic quadriplegia
Ataxic/hypotonia
Athetosis/dyskinesia
Mixed types

backs, namely (1) the changing nature of the clinical signs in an individual over time, and (2) clinicians applying differing interpretations to the terms used in description of the signs. This variability in definition makes comparison of statistics from different centres difficult, and is a major problem in epidemiological research. Some progress has been made recently in achieving a broadly acceptable yet precise method of clinical description (Evans and Alberman, 1985).

In our centre, and in this book, classification is based upon the clinical neurological syndrome, without regard to aetiology. This classification is limited to the major groupings in general usage and each category, and is, therefore, very broad (Table 1.2).

1.2.1   HEMIPLEGIA

In this condition most children present with spastic weakness which is unilateral. There may be associated seizures (25%) and learning difficulties. Athetoid movement in the affected side may be prominent.

1.2.2   DIPLEGIA AND ATAXIC DIPLEGIA

It is recognized that these two syndromes are clinically and aetiologically quite different, but in both conditions arm involvement is relatively minor, and the major clinical signs present in the lower limbs and hips. We do not use the term paraplegia for those children who have no discernible arm involvement. Such children require very careful evaluation, because in these cases a progressive spinal lesion must be excluded. Static spinal lesions have been described in children with cerebral palsy (Harrison, 1988).

1.2.3   QUADRIPLEGIA OR TOTAL BODY INVOLVEMENT

In this condition there is four-limb spasticity associated with truncal, cephalic and oral facial difficulties. In our centre this term is also used to describe children who have double hemiplegia. This is an essentially pragmatic usage, as most children with total body involvement have asymmetries, and we have not found it possible to make a useful division of these cases. Learning difficulties and epilepsy are frequently additional handicaps in these children.

1.2.4 ATAXIA/HYPOTONIA

In this condition, the muscle tone is diminished and ataxia during volitional movement is present. Dysmetria (past pointing) and problems with limb speed (dysdiadochokinesia) are usually present.

1.2.5 ATHETOSIS DYSKINESIA

In these children the predominant features include the incoordinate generalized movement which occurs during volitional movement. Tone may fluctuate, and dystonia may be present (fluctuation between normal and increased tone).

1.2.6 MIXED TYPES

In some children the motor disorder may be difficult to classify into the above groups. Tone may be variable but be predominantly spastic, and athetosis may not be dominant. Varying degrees of ataxia may be seen, particularly in the very young child.

The hypotonic child with severe learning difficulties, who presents with global developmental delay, and in whom motor functional development is retarded, is not classified as having cerebral palsy in our centre, but rather as having a global developmental delay. The children in this group most often progress to develop independent mobility and in most cases there is not a recognizable structural brain lesion, and there is usually a recovery of muscle tone in the long term.

1.3 Terminology

A variety of terms is used to describe the clinical features of children with cerebral palsy, and it may be useful at this stage to review the meanings of these terms as they appear later in the book.

Hypertonia refers to increased resistance to passive movement of the limb. There is usually an associated increase in deep tendon reflexes in the affected limb.

Hypotonia implies decreased muscle tone. The muscles are soft and floppy, and there is usually increased joint range. Deep tendon reflexes may be diminished, or may be normal or exaggerated.

Spasticity: muscle tone is persistently increased, with abnormal resistance to passive movement, which may be associated with the clasp-knife phenomenon. It is associated with increased deep tendon reflexes and frequently fluctuates with posture.

Rigidity implies sustained increase in muscle tone with the characteristic of 'lead pipe'.

Ataxia implies excessive incoordination of voluntary movement for the patient's age. Most obviously this is manifest in the arm and hand skills, but also gross body movements may be affected, e.g. head and trunk control, and gait. It may be associated with nystagmus and hypotonia, and is often symptomatic of a cerebellar lesion.

Athetosis: athetoid movement is movement extraneous to the desired task, usually of a slow, writhing character. There is an excessive recruitment of inappropriate muscle groups during the activity.

Dystonia: this refers to fluctuating tone, in which the child's muscle tone is usually normal or increased, infrequently decreased.

1.4   Prevalence

Prevalence of a condition is the number of cases of the disorder existing in the population at a given time. It is clearly important, when reporting the prevalence of cerebral palsy, to define the denominator population (i.e. whether birth cohort, 3-year-old, or school age). However, in spite of methodological variations, most surveys give a prevalence of cerebral palsy in the order of 2 per 1000 (Stanley and Alberman, 1984).

Variations in reported prevalence of cerebral palsy can broadly be reduced to three main origins.

1. Variability in definition, for example whether those cases of a postnatal aetiology are included.
2. Analysis of service usage or population study or cohort follow-up, all render a different ascertainment of positive cases. (For example, there is an increased rate of diagnosis in cohort follow-up studies, particularly with reference to mild cases.)
3. Changes with time. Most post-war studies have suggested a relatively constant prevalence of cerebral palsy in Western countries, but recent reports suggest there may be an increasing prevalence over the past ten years (Pharoah *et al.*, 1987). The impact of improved neonatal care on the prevalence of cerebral palsy is a question which is yet to be resolved. Some authors conclude that an increased

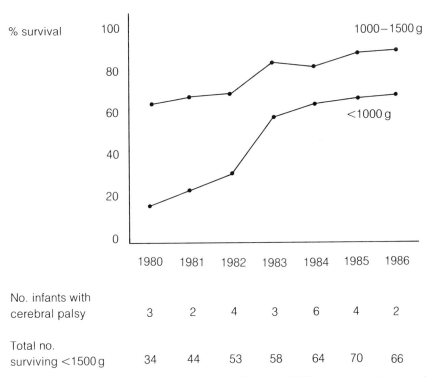

Fig. 1.2 Survival of low birth weight infants (<1500 g) and incidence of cerebral palsy, Sheffield Health District 1980–6.

incidence of cerebral palsy has been due to the increased survival of extremely low birth weight infants (Brown, 1984). In our own experience this seems not to be the case. The great improvements in survival of extremely low birth weight infants born within the Sheffield Health District between 1980 and 1986 was not associated with any significant increase in the prevalence of cerebral palsy. Figure 1.2 demonstrates the changes in mortality for two weight groups over the period 1980–6, with the follow-up data on survivors from these groups. These figures are representative of a defined population in which population drift is very small (less than 3% per annum).

1.5 Aetiology

The understanding of some of the aetiological mechanisms in cerebral palsy has been advanced by the recent application of improved imaging techniques. Computerized axial tomography and particularly neonatal cerebral ultrasonography have given considerable insight into the nature and evolution of cerebral haemorrhagic and ischaemic lesions, and their long-term consequences. Exciting new developments in magnetic resonance imaging (McArdle *et al.*, 1987) and spectroscopy (Wyatt *et al.*, 1989), near infrared spectroscopy (Edwards *et al.*, 1989) and positron emission tomography (Volpe *et al.*, 1983) have advanced our understanding of the metabolic and developmental features of brain injury and will expand our knowledge of these disorders during the coming decade.

1.5.1 HEMIPLEGIA

It is now known that the majority of infants with hemiplegia have a lesion in the distribution of the middle cerebral artery in the hemisphere contralateral to the spastic weakness. It has been possible to deduce the timing of onset of these lesions from recently developed imaging techniques. Larroche and Amiel (1966) observed that infarction of cerebral tissue in early fetal life resulted in cortical neuronal loss and appearances of polymicrogyria, presumably secondary to disruption of neuronal migration (Norman, 1980). Lesions occurring later in gestation are associated with the development of cavitatory changes. The role of embolization in the genesis of cerebral artery infarction is not yet clear. It has been postulated that the association of hemiplegia with smallness for dates, placental infarction or repeated bleeding in pregnancy, implies the presence of either placental microemboli or polycythaemia. Either secondary condition may lead to luminal vascular obstruction in the middle cerebral artery and hence hemiplegia. In Hagberg's series, 45 of 200 cases of hemiplegia (Hagberg *et al.*, 1975) were associated with smallness for dates, placental infarction or repeated bleeding. Cocker, George and Yates (1965) reported pathological studies in two children in whom organizing thrombus was identified in the middle cerebral artery. Similar findings were reported by Clark and Linnell (1954) and Banker (1961).

Middle cerebral artery infarction may come about as a consequence of perinatal asphyxia (Brown *et al.*, 1974; Hagberg *et al.*, 1975). Infarction may follow hypoxia and hypoperfusion, intraluminal obstruction in these cases seeming much less likely. In 41% of Hagberg's series of hemiplegia, the cause was thought to be perinatal asphyxia. Brown (1974), reporting outcome following severe birth asphyxia, recorded 7 of 42 handicapped survivors as hemiplegic.

In preterm infants, hemiplegia may develop as a consequence of haemorrhagic and/or ischaemic lesions which are peculiar to this period of development. Haemorrhagic ischaemic involvement, wherein

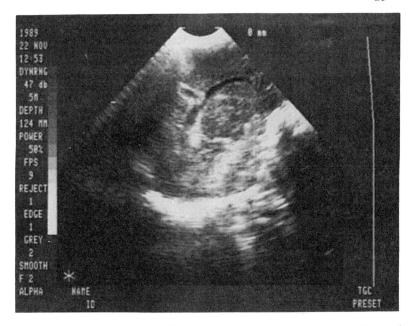

Fig. 1.3 Parasagittal cranial ultrasound scan of 29 weeks' gestation infant showing left-sided haemorrhagic intracerebral infarction breaking down to form a cyst. This child developed a right hemiplegia.

the periventricular white matter becomes infarcted and haemorrhagic, may be followed by the later development of a single cyst with an associated contralateral hemiparesis. The aetiology of this condition is not yet clear. Data from pathological specimens (Pape and Wigglesworth, 1979) and from positron emission tomography (Volpe *et al.*, 1983) suggest this lesion occurs as a result of venous infarction. In our series of four preterm infants who developed hemiplegia, three demonstrated haemorrhagic intracerebral involvement; the fourth was not scanned in the neonatal period (Fig. 1.3).

Postnatal stroke may also occur due to infection (meningitis/ventriculitis) (Hagberg and Hagberg, 1984; Ment *et al.*, 1984), and in association with exchange transfusion (Hagberg and Hagberg, 1984). In a number of cases a precise aetiological description will not be possible due to an absence of any pre-, peri- or postnatal risk factor (30.5% of Hagberg's series, 50% of Sheffield cases).

1.5.2 SPASTIC DIPLEGIA

Spastic diplegia is most frequently associated with low birth weight (Davies and Tizard, 1975; Powell *et al.*, 1988). The classic lesion associated with the later development of spastic diplegia is periventricular leucomalacia. This condition occurs predominantly between 24 and 36 weeks' gestation. The term refers to white matter necrosis in the area adjacent to the external angles of the lateral cerebral ventricles. Banker and Larroche (1962) described the pathological development of this lesion. Neuronal necrosis occurs; this may be associated with haemorrhage (Armstrong and Norman, 1974) and, in some cases, the later development of cystic cavities. It is now widely accepted that this lesion develops as a result of impaired cerebral perfusion, the predilection for this site resulting from the characteristics of the cerebral circulation at this period in gestation. Periventricular leucomalacia (PVL) arises in areas which are arterial border zones or end zones (Volpe, 1981). Also the preterm infant is particularly susceptible to underperfusion of these areas due to the limited capacity for cerebrovascular autoregulation (Lou *et al.*, 1979).

It has been appreciated that periventricular leucomalacia can be recognized in the neonatal period using real time ultrasonography (Levene *et al.*, 1983). Later studies (e.g. Bozynski *et al.*, 1988) have demonstrated the association of cavitatory PVL with the later development of spastic diplegia.

In the 12 preterm cases of spastic diplegia in the Sheffield series, five had cavitatory PVL in the neonatal period. Two infants had intraventricular haemorrhage followed by post-haemorrhagic hydrocephalus requiring shunt placement, one infant suffered hypoxic ischaemic encephalopathy without cavitatory changes, two children in the early years of the study were not scanned.

In term infants who develop spastic diplegia, there may be a history of perinatal asphyxia, particularly in the infant who is small for dates (Alberman, 1963). In such cases the children usually display other neuro-developmental problems such as specific or global learning defects, epilepsy, or visual disorders (Veelken *et al.*, 1983). A small number of children with spastic diplegia have genetically determined disease, which may be autosomal dominant, autosomal recessive or sex-linked.

1.5.3   SPASTIC QUADRIPLEGIA

The aetiology of spastic quadriplegia is perhaps even more heterogeneous than the preceding forms.

In our series of 46 cases of quadriplegia (Table 1.3) there was a large number of cases of undefinable cause. No peri- or postnatal factors could be identified and the cause is presumably prenatal in these cases. In their review of the antecedents of cerebral palsy, Nelson and

Table 1.3 Aetiology of cerebral palsy – Sheffield Health District

Hemiplegia	28	4 prematurity
		3 term asphyxia
		21 prenatal
Diplegia	24	12 prematurity
		1 term asphyxia
		11 prenatal
Quadriplegia	46	7 prematurity
		8 term asphyxia
		31 prenatal
Ataxia/hypotonia	5	2 posterior fossa malformation
		3 unknown

Ellenberg (1986) refer to such aetiological problems; in the present state of knowledge there are many cases where 'we simply do not know the cause'.

In the Sheffield series a small number of children had definite prenatal causes; four children with major primary CNS malformation. In one case in this group, the initial presumption was that perinatal asphyxia was causative but CT scan established the diagnosis of lobar holoprosencephaly. In this case the primary cerebral malformation had presumably rendered the infant more susceptible to the effects of labour and delivery. A similar malformation was described by Shanks and Wilson (1988) in association with spastic diplegia.

Other prenatal influences which may be associated with the development of quadriplegic cerebral palsy include maternal trauma (Ferrer and Navarro, 1978); monozygotic twinning (Aicardi and Goutieres, 1972; Smith and Rodeck, 1975), in which the second twin is small, stillborn and often macerated, while the first develops multicystic encephalomalacia. It is possible that cerebral damage occurs as a result of direct passage of material from the circulation of the dead fetus into the survivor. We have seen similar CT appearances in singleton survivors of severe perinatal asphyxia (Fig. 1.4). Other causative factors include fetal viral infection with cytomegalovirus (Hagberg and Hagberg, 1984), rubella and possibly mumps (Lyen *et al.*, 1981); fetal toxoplasmosis; and fetal cerebral haemorrhage in association with thrombocytopenia (Jesurum *et al.*, 1980) or maternal drug administration (Robinson *et al.*, 1980).

In our view, and with the benefit of many recent studies, the aetiological role of perinatal asphyxia in spastic quadriplegia can only be sustained when there has been a significant post-asphyxial encephalopathy. Other indices of perinatal asphyxia such as Apgar score and

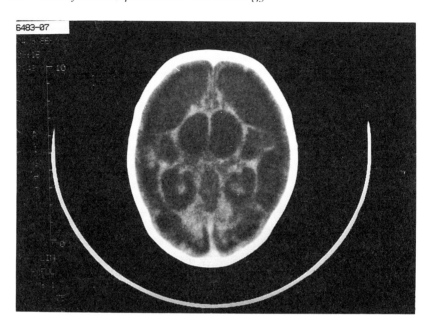

Fig. 1.4 Cerebral computerized tomographic scan showing multicystic encephalomalacia. Term infant age 3 months, severe perinatal asphyxia.

umbilical arterial pH at birth, are only weakly associated with later adverse outcome (Nelson and Ellenberg, 1981; Levene *et al.*, 1986). From 1980 to 1985 we studied all infants with a 5-minute Apgar score below 7. Thirty-nine infants entered the study, but only those infants who developed Stage II or III post-asphyxial hypoxic ischaemic encephalopathy (HIE) were at risk of subsequent cerebral palsy. Sarnat and Sarnat (1976) described the features of Stages I, II and III HIE. In their study, all infants in Stage I recovered completely and were normal at follow-up, whereas infants who developed Stage II were at high risk of cerebral palsy, and all infants in Stage III either died or were severely impaired. In their larger study of follow-up of HIE at 3.5 years, Robertson and Finer (1985) reported all infants who developed Stage I to be normal, 23% of Stage II HIE to be handicapped, and all Stage III children to be handicapped. Of the handicapped survivors, 52.6% had cerebral palsy, the commonest form being spastic quadriplegia.

All the infants who developed spastic quadriplegia in association with preterm birth in the 1980–5 series developed severe cerebral disorders in association with other neonatal illnesses.

1.5.4 ATAXIA HYPOTONIA

In this group of conditions, genetic factors seem to be most important. In the five cases in this group, two had recessively inherited posterior fossa malformations in association with retinal dystrophy (one with alternating tachypnoea and apnoea – Joubert syndrome). In the series of Hagberg and Hagberg (1984) hereditary features were found to be the most important single aetiological characteristic. Perinatal risk factors were no more commonly represented in this group of ataxic children than within the general population, and these authors stressed the importance of recessively inherited syndromes in children with ataxia and learning difficulties. Gustavson *et al.* (1969) described ten families with two or more affected members with congenital ataxia and learning difficulties.

1.5.5 DYSKINETIC SYNDROMES

While we observe a number of children who have a primarily dyskinetic syndrome from our regional practice, we did not see a new case of primarily dyskinetic cerebral palsy between 1980 and 1986 from the local health district. These disorders are particularly associated with postnatal brain damage, as a result of hyperbilirubinaemia (Ingram, 1964) due to rhesus disease or associated with prematurity. The second major causative factor is perinatal asphyxia (Hagberg and Hagberg, 1984). However, the predominant handicap in the Sheffield infants (1980–6) who had severe hypoxic ischaemic encephalopathy was spastic quadriplegia, usually in association with global learning difficulties.

PART TWO
Development and Cerebral Palsy

Introduction

The chapters in Part Two trace the development of a person with cerebral palsy from babyhood to young adulthood.

Using normal development and society's expectations as reference points, the tasks required of the child and his or her family at each significant stage are outlined. These tasks may be physical or intellectual or involve adjustment by the family to the evolving handicap.

Reference is also made to relationships between the child, family and health and education services.

2 The baby

2.1 Family issues

2.1.1 PARENTAL ADJUSTMENT

It is not known when parents begin to construct a mental image of the expected child. The image has its origins in the parents' own childhood and is influenced by their lifestyle and expectations. During pregnancy the image becomes more sharply defined and expectations of the child's physical appearance develop. Expectations of the child's achievement may extend into the future (for example, scholastic performance). When the infant is delivered early or presents with serious illness in the newborn period, these expectations are threatened. The idea of a healthy, contented baby is replaced by the reality of a sick newborn whose survival may be in doubt and around whom there is a lot of medical activity. The separation from the child and the difficulty in comprehending the nature of the medical problems increase the stress on parents. The evolution of a cerebral disorder in these circumstances, with the associated risk of subsequent handicap, comes as a further disturbing event. The parents' expectations have been disturbed and they will be anxious and extremely sensitive to the child's subsequent development.

The parental adjustment to the presence of cerebral palsy in the child has important differences from the process seen where the child has a recognizable handicap from birth (e.g. Down's syndrome). There is a need for a period of observation in order to confirm or refute the diagnosis and this is an additional stress on parents in an already difficult situation. In one sense the presence of a recognizable and well-documented disorder is easier to accommodate because the immediate diagnostic certainty at least allows confidence in the disclosure and broad assessment of prognosis. In contrast the evolving early physical signs and symptoms in cerebral palsy gradually confirm the parents' fears. We need to recognize this attenuated adaptation process and be sensitive to the parents' feelings during it.

2.1.2   DIAGNOSIS

The reactions of the parents will be importantly influenced by the way in which the child's problem presents and by the way in which discussions about diagnosis and prognosis are undertaken. The recognition of cerebral palsy may arise in one of three ways.

(a)   During follow-up of an 'at risk' infant

In approximately half the cases of cerebral palsy in our series (Chapter 1) the child had presented with a perinatal illness which placed the child at risk of later cerebral palsy. As a result, some discussion was possible with the parents from the outset. The objective of the development review was explained and the parents' questions answered with respect to the degree of risk. In cases where deviant neurological signs persisted beyond the first week in association with morphological cerebral anomalies ('bright brain', periventricular cysts, multicystic encephalomalacia), the subsequent presentation of cerebral palsy was extremely common. The outcome for a child presenting with transient periventricular echo-density, single cysts or transient generalized echo-density, was more variable.

Parents must in these cases be given the fullest information, but professionals and parents alike have to accept a period of observation and doubt before accurate diagnosis can be achieved. Particular difficulty is experienced in cases in which there is a 'mild' abnormality on ultrasound/computerized scan in a child with minor neurological signs. It may be many months in these cases before resolution of the doubt can be achieved.

(b)   During routine screening/examination for other illness

In these cases the parents may or may not have suspected a problem. The paediatrician is here in a very difficult situation, as it may not be possible to make a definite diagnosis and it may be necessary to seek further advice from colleagues. In these circumstances, we have found it most helpful to describe the deviant development and the need for developmental therapy and further investigation.

It is important to recognize that diagnosis of a specific syndrome may not be possible and this difficulty should be fully explained to the family.

(c)   Parental anxiety about the child's progress

In these cases there is a high frequency of parents' recognition of a problem in their child but difficulty is found in convincing others of it. There is a professional reluctance to make a firm statement in diagnosis, given the changing clinical nature of the disorder. In management of these situations it is important to recognize parents' fears and deal with them rather than denying the source of anxiety and giving reassurance. Again, it is possible to describe a feature in development as deviant without necessarily resorting to diagnosis of cerebral palsy, and in this description to the parents one can introduce the notion of developmental therapy which can commence before the firm diagnosis is established. Too often we meet families where therapy has been delayed until a definite diagnostic statement has been made. This is unnecessary. Honest, detailed discussion at each stage in the evolution of the problem is found to be satisfactory to most parents.

2.1.3 DISCLOSURE

In discussing parental reaction to disclosure, we must again consider parental expectations of the child. McKeith (1973) drew attention to the common parental reactions to diagnosis of a handicapping condition in their child. He described five aspects:

1. Biological reactions, for example, protection of the helpless child or revulsion at the abnormality.
2. Inadequacy, for example, at reproductive capacity, especially if the child is the first child: feelings of inadequacy related to the parents' inability to manage the situation.
3. Bereavement: shock, anger, grief at the loss of the normal child.
4. Embarrassment: e.g. public acceptance and acceptance by the extended family.
5. Guilt at one's own feelings: for example of rejection and revulsion, or, in view of the feeling of parental responsibility towards the child, a feeling of responsibility for 'creating' the problem.

Cunningham and Davis (1985) added the following:

6. Feelings of fear of the future, uncertainty of the outcome, fear of death of the child, fear of feelings towards the child and fear of attachment.

We may find that the disclosure comes as a relief to some parents, as it focuses months of doubt and suspicion and helps them understand the child's problem and allows them to reconstrue the future.

Many of these reactions are common in parents of newly diagnosed children with disability. It is important to recognize that all parents are not the same and within the pair there may be widely different feelings about the child's problem. Feelings change with time, and part of the adaptation process is an integration of the above reactions to diagnosis. As parents begin to adapt to the new circumstances and seek help in dealing with the problem, there may be times when their thoughts and feelings return to the early reactions following disclosure. It is not uncommon for parents to describe and discuss such feelings, sometimes many years after the problem is recognized. We must also consider that the evolution of subsequent problems (for example, hearing loss, visual defect, learning difficulty) within the primary disability may have similar effects upon the parents.

These disclosures require equally sensitive management, discussion and parental support. As the parents start to adapt to the diagnosis, we consider their adaptation and ability to cope with the child and the handicap. It is important to appreciate that coping or adaptation is only a temporary circumstance; parents try to deal with current problems and reconstrue the future. As the child grows and develops, however, further adaptation has to be accomplished: the recognition, for example, of the differences presented by their child and the average 2-year-old; the appreciation of associated developmental problems such as speech delay; later issues over educational needs and school placement have to be accommodated and many more issues throughout the growth and development of the individual. Related to this is the area of professional as opposed to parental perception of problems. As professionals we need to remind ourselves that the recognition of what we see as additional though minor developmental problems may produce severe reactions in the parents, similar to those described at disclosure. In some cases the parents' perception of the problem may be that the individual problem is minor but the cumulative effect of so many difficulties can be overwhelming. Therefore, we need to apply the same degree of care and consideration in discussing these problems as we do at the earlier phase of the process.

Further discussion of the principles of working with families follows in Chapter 3, on the early years.

2.2 Moving and manipulation

The movement patterns of babies have been observed *in utero* as early as 9 weeks' gestation. Sucking and swallowing as well as isolated head, leg and arm movements have been described by deVries (1984). These activities are considered necessary for later muscle and joint development, but they take place within an environment which is largely free from the effects of gravity. The newly born infant suddenly has to cope with this new and overwhelming force.

Orientating head movements with respect to gravity is particularly difficult, and this is one of the major tasks of the first few months. Until the head and body can overcome gravity, the baby will continue to require a lot of physical support. During the first six months she learns to control her head in most positions and enjoys being propped in sitting. Her head is fully erect, and she is able to look around and reach out for desired objects.

When the baby first tries to sit alone, she easily topples over if she reaches out too far. In the space of a few months, balance reactions become more skilful and accurate. There is, in effect, an increased control of the forces of gravity. The baby will then be able, for example, to twist around when sitting and retrieve a toy behind her. If someone tries to push her sideways her body will tilt appropriately, thus keeping her upright. If her position is further threatened, however, and the tilt reaction is not enough to resist this force, the baby will fall over. Alternatively, she may have learnt to catch her weight by reaching out her arm.

Towards the end of the first year, the infant starts to crawl, pull to stand and cruise around furniture. These tasks require a highly developed postural control and, at least initially, much concentration. This is also true of rolling, creeping, crawling and bottom-shuffling. When the infant first walks alone, her arms are held out to the side, and her face reflects the difficulty of this emerging skill. The child's balance is easily disturbed, and there need to be well coordinated muscular adaptations if she is not to fall.

The balancing skills required for sitting, standing and walking develop during the first year, and they become more refined during childhood. The maintenance of balance requires the integration of information from many sensory systems (tactile, proprioceptive, visual, vestibular), and it is the basis of all coordinated and efficient movement.

The speed of motor progress is influenced by many factors, and there is a wide variability in the age at which motor milestones may be reached. The infant born very prematurely and nursed predominantly in extended postures may show an early prowess with supported standing, but be delayed with sitting balance. Other factors such as body structure, sex, neural maturation, environment and motivation may influence motor progress.

These factors may also influence manipulative abilities. The newborn infant usually grasps objects placed in her palm in an automatic way. In the next few months, manipulation becomes more deliberate; the baby is able to hold a rattle and wave it around. During the latter part of the first year the grasping patterns become more coordinated. The older baby is able to pick up small crumbs between the thumb and index finger. This sophisticated control of fingers develops in the first year.

2.2.1 LOCOMOTION AND MANIPULATION IN THE BABY WITH CEREBRAL PALSY

Movement is an integral part of the overall development of the infant and child. Delay or abnormality of any aspect of motor development may have widespread or cumulative effects on a child's overall development. The child with cerebral palsy has abnormalities of tone, posture and movement which affect her ability to experience and explore her world. For example, the baby who has difficulty developing head control will have difficulty developing in many other areas. She will have difficulty rolling, sitting alone, controlling her gaze and feeding.

This is particularly true of the child with quadriplegia. She may lie with her head consistently turned to the side, and some of the automatic reactions usually seen in babies will continue to be present in an obligatory way. The asymmetric neck reaction (straightening the arm on the side to which the head turns) is particularly problematic as it interferes with the ability to bring hands to the middle for play.

The baby who has hemiplegia (i.e. with a poverty of leg and arm movements on one side) may not have particular difficulty with lifting the head, but will be unwilling to roll because of difficulties coordinating the affected limbs. When reaching for toys the child will usually do this with the more coordinated arm and hand; the other hand may be fisted and held close to the body. The baby who has less severe problems may be able to hold a rattle if it is deliberately placed in the affected hand. However, movements may be jerky, and often the mouth is used instead of the other hand to explore a toy.

Babies with diplegia tend to find it difficult to sit without help. They are unable to open their legs far enough to give a sufficiently wide base of support and easily topple over if they take their hands away. They therefore find it difficult to play in sitting and often prefer to lie on their backs so that their hands are released and able to hold a toy.

Usually children need little encouragement to achieve independence in movement. They will enjoy moving and repeat activities many times during the day. With increasing strength, balance and coordination, the motor skills become more refined. The child with cerebral palsy has more difficulty enjoying movement and will therefore either refrain from the full range of activities or repeat poor, or even damaging, patterns of movement.

2.2.2   PARENT AND PROFESSIONAL TASKS

All motor development is influenced by environmental opportunities, motivation and encouragement, and this is especially true for the child with cerebral palsy. We have looked exclusively at movement problems, but it is important to recognize that limitations of movement are intertwined with cognitive, emotional and communicative factors. Parents and professionals alike tend to focus primarily on motor factors at the expense of these other areas, and this is particularly true during the first years of life. However, the parents need a good understanding of their child's physical problems so that they can help their child learn to move and explore. The parents also need to appreciate their child's physical signals so that the child is not unduly frustrated. For example, a fisted hand lifted a little from the body may be the child's only way of indicating a preference when offered a choice of toys.

In order to maximize the child's interaction with her environment it may be necessary to use adapted seating or specialized equipment. Once the child has achieved a stable position, she will find it easier to look around and to use her hands for play (see Chapter 10 on seating).

It is important that the carer should have a clear understanding of how to encourage opportunities for broadening the movement repertoire, and conversely, how to discourage undesirable movement patterns. Any child will need time to experiment with movement and manipulation, but the child with cerebral palsy will need both more time and adult assistance. The child may need to put in a great deal of effort to complete a task, and if that effort is not rewarded the child may understandably give up and avoid the task in future.

2.3   Communication

2.3.1   THE DEVELOPMENT OF INTERACTION

The baby's first task is to ensure continuing care. Eibl-Eibesfeldt (1970) has suggested that the young of any species requiring special parenting have to ensure that such parenting is forthcoming. He introduced the idea of 'babyness' – a relatively large head, large forehead in relation to the rest of the face, large, low-set eyes, etc. – as a set of features which triggers caring behaviours in the adult. These behaviours include social interaction. Daniel Stern (1977) maintains that 'a strong tendency exists in the vast majority of us to respond in a fairly stereotypic and predictable way' to the sight of a baby, although he stresses that the behaviours are not always evoked and that there is a wide variability in response.

Interaction with a baby usually involves exaggerated facial expressions and bizarre pitch changes, which hold the baby's attention and maximize learning. Stern calls these adult behaviours 'infant elicited social behaviours'.

With the development of the smile and its potent effects on adult behaviour, opportunities arise for the baby to learn such communicative prerequisites as turntaking and cause and effect. The baby also learns about initiating, responding to and maintaining social interaction, in that the smile firstly signals a readiness to interact, then that an interaction is going well, and, in the event of a breakdown, a desire to re-engage in the interaction.

Babies are also predisposed to look at faces (Fantz, 1966); their principal interest being in the eyes and mouth. This predisposition helps the baby to learn that important messages are sent by the face and that by using eye contact she can attract and hold the attention of adults. Joint attention and reference have their roots in the early months when parents watch the direction of the baby's eyes and reinforce the interest by moving the object closer and/or talking about it. Eye contact and eye 'pointing' thus rapidly become meaningful and communicative. The baby's appearance, smile and eye contact are thus all significant factors in the development of interactional skills.

(a)   The implications of physical disability for the development of interaction

The baby who spends time in a Special Care Baby Unit or other hospital setting is often attached to equipment that physically prevents, or at least discourages, parents from holding the baby and having an active role in care of the child. The opportunities for developing communicative rhythm may be further hindered by the very fact of the baby's illness and the parents' helplessness and grief in the face of it.

The baby with cerebral palsy may have hypertonia to a degree where attempts at action will cause extensor thrusting. Even a smile in response to the sight of a face will cause the baby's whole body to exhibit an extensor pattern such that the head will tip back and the eyes roll upwards, thus losing (visual) contact with the original stimulus. Lacking the appropriate feedback, the 'face' may move away and the baby will have failed to respond to and maintain a social interaction. A blank, or mistimed, response may have the same result and turntaking is therefore very difficult to establish.

Similarly, the baby's attempts to locate objects of interest may be thwarted by poor head and eye control. The parents will consequently not find it easy or natural to interpret these attempts, and opportunities to learn joint attention are missed.

2.3.2 HEARING AND LISTENING

In the normal parent – baby dyad, close physical contact, together with the rhythm and voice produced by rocking and soothing, provides the baby with an integrated sensory input: sound is part of a pleasurable activity to which the baby is alert. Later, when location of sound begins, the baby's visual search for a sound source is frequently rewarded by interaction with a person. Listening ability is a major factor in attracting the baby's attention and maintaining interest in events in the environment.

Research suggests that very young babies are able to discriminate many of the essential basics of the characteristics of speech sounds (Eimas, 1974), and logically they are able to segment the speech stream into words.

There is a primary risk of a hearing loss co-occurring with the cerebral palsy (see section 7.1 on hearing assessment).

Even in babies with measurably normal hearing, however, secondary problems may arise. The sick baby or the baby who is awkward to hold due to tone abnormalities, may not be cuddled and spoken to as frequently as would normally be expected. Some authorities (e.g. Holt and Reynell, 1967) feel that this deprivation of auditory stimulation can lead to delayed development of hearing.

Impaired development of head control leads to great difficulty in the localization of sound source. This leads to reduced motivation and thereby reduced experience.

2.3.3 DEVELOPMENT OF LANGUAGE UNDERSTANDING

Early experience of the human voice in pleasurable situations helps the baby to attune to language. Voice is calming and through the association of language with everyday situations, the baby becomes familiar with commonly used words and phrases. Baby games and songs help the infant to learn rhythm and anticipation of events which become associated with language.

The major implication of physical handicap for language understanding is that of reduced experience. As with hearing development, auditory awareness and interest in voice stem from close physical contact with parents who talk and sing to the baby. The baby's physical condition, whether illness-related or postural, may preclude this. Cuddling may seem to distress the baby, and anxious or depressed parents may find it difficult to entertain the baby naturally.

Knowledge of the world is vital for language development, and the immobile baby is at a disadvantage.

2.3.4   EXPRESSING LANGUAGE

Understanding develops in close reciprocity with expression. The baby's sounds and gestures encourage interaction from adults and evidence that the baby *can* understand such as 'byebye' or clapping in 'pat-a-cake' leads adults to expect and try to elicit yet more. The baby who is restricted physically may be slow to respond, may not respond at all, or may make physical responses that are not recognized as being appropriate.

For a child with cerebral palsy, the implications of tone abnormalities which affect the muscle groups required to make fine, sequenced, rapid movements, are enormous. In severe spastic quadriplegia, the *possible* range of mouth movements may be so limited as to render coordinated voice and articulation for rapid speech unlikely.

In the baby with cerebral palsy, the voluntary vocalization that begins at 6 weeks may not occur, voice production being affected by poor head control and posture. Vocalization may be involuntary and associated with extensor thrusting. Conversely, attempts at vocalization may cause tonal reactions and target sounds cannot be achieved. Babies with poor control over their voluntary movements either through excessive involuntary movement or hypotonia will have difficulty in approximating the articulators and will lack experience in producing sounds. This has implications for praxis and also for the acquisition of a phonological system.

Disordered oral sensation may occur and be compounded by the lack of experience in mouthing if the baby is unable to bring toys to the mouth.

Using speech in a communicative act requires accuracy and timing, skills usually learned in the baby stage through babble, imitation and interactive games. Babies also use body posture, gaze and facial expression to augment their speech attempts. The baby whose intention to communicate is hampered by physical disability may experience frustration when her communication attempts are misinterpreted.

2.3.5   PARENT AND PROFESSIONAL TASKS

The parents' role is to open up two-way communication with the baby, ensuring the maximum quality of input and opportunity for output. Cerebral palsy affects the development of this communication in the baby by disrupting the natural sequence of patterns of interaction. The lack of confidence this can cause in the parents compounds communication difficulties, in as much as they may feel more comfortable dealing with the baby's physical needs at the expense of providing valuable interaction experiences for the baby.

Their confidence may be further undermined by insensitive

therapeutic intervention which fails to take account of the parent/child relationship. Therapists should take care not to monopolize the child and thereby exclude the parents. It is communication patterns peculiar to the parent/baby dyad, and not those between the therapist and baby, which should be fostered.

The great value of assessment of the activities of daily living is in generating new ideas for ameliorating disability and in providing the professionals with the information needed to assist the person with disability to make informed choices. Communication patterns are peculiar to the parent – baby dyad and it is these patterns and not those between the therapist and baby which should be fostered.

The professionals involved with the family should try to determine the existing interaction between parents and baby and, most importantly, how the parents construe that interaction in terms of successful, enjoyable, and so on.

(a) Intention

Perhaps the most powerful factor in the development of communication is the interpretation of intent, even if, as in a very young baby, that intent does not exist. Interpretation allows the interaction to be spontaneous and child-led and teaches turn-taking, contingency, timing and joint attention, as well as specific verbal and non-verbal representations of the world.

Understanding and expressive language can develop in a social context as the baby learns that certain behaviours lead to a predictable outcome. This helps to bring the behaviour under voluntary control.

Exercise of control in communication is vital and regularly occurring behaviours in the baby make adults more likely to interact and provide linguistic information. The professional may be able to help redirect the parents towards interpretation of intent. As well as offering support, the professionals can help the parents to recognize possibly minute changes in behaviour, which can be interpreted as meaningful.

The questions which may be used in assessment to gather information for the professional may heighten the parents' awareness of their baby's communicative behaviours, for example, how does the baby let you know she is hungry, tired, in need of a cuddle?

(b) Getting the right position

An important factor in enabling the child to have maximum contact with people is positioning. The best position is one that allows the child full eye contact while at the same time stabilizing the head and shoulders, to allow purposeful vocalization and oral movement. Also desirable is some freedom for the baby to change position in the room, for example, by being carried so that she can choose with whom she communicates. Interaction during cuddling should be encouraged as babies frequently interact at 'mother distance'; when cradled in an adult's arms so that the body is fully supported, the eyes are at an optimal focal distance from the adult's face and the baby can see the source of voice.

(c)   Listening and understanding

'Physical and mental handicap dominate the clinical picture and in many cases once deafness has been excluded, little attention is paid to the subsequent development of hearing. This is a mistake because hearing development is ultimately linked with emotional and speech development' (Holt and Reynell, 1967).

The professionals involved with the baby should aim to keep hearing in the forefront. Continuous assessment will be necessary, and the information and its implications passed to the parents and other professionals. It is important not only to test the level and pattern of hearing but also the quality of the baby's response to sound. Responses will change over time and continued dissemination of results is vital. In the area of hearing and listening support for the parents is crucial. Their feelings of guilt, anxiety and disbelief, together with the knowledge that the baby can hear may discourage them from extra effort in providing auditory experience. The professionals can provide information, ideas, and perhaps some motivation for prolonged, conscious auditory input to the child. The baby will need good quality auditory input and help to orientate her face towards the sound source. Songs and routines in addition to relevant language input are important for the baby, as they provide repetition and regularity on which to base expectations so that understanding of language can develop.

Professionals can join with the parents in continuous assessment of the baby's progress in understanding to ensure that appropriate input is given to the baby.

(d)   Making sounds and talking

At the baby stage, the parents' role is to encourage the development of communication by any means available to the baby. Babies with physical difficulties may not be able to produce the finely organized movements necessary for voice production (eye contact, eye pointing, body gesture). The parents, therefore, are put in a position of having to interpret a range of movements or vocalizations around a target as having meaning. Vocalization, voluntary or otherwise, can be interpreted as having meaning. This should increase the likelihood of subsequent utterances and provide the baby with further targets. In the baby stage, most communication is child-led, but with the baby with severe physical disability, the parents' role may be much more active and leading. Parents have to be aware of this while remaining open to the baby's communication attempts.

2.4 Seeing and perceiving

2.4.1 DEVELOPMENT OF VISION

The newborn baby is optically well equipped but immature. The focal length of vision is approximately 25 cm, but the baby can see movement and brightness at a greater distance. The infant makes gross orientations towards a source of visual stimulation; she looks at faces and face-like shapes and complex visual patterns (Fantz, 1966) and she converges on an object and tracks it through 180° (Forfar and Arneil, 1984).

By 4 months the baby can distinguish a familiar face and locate and track objects, reach out and grasp them. In the second half of this first year, the mobile baby can move towards that which is visually interesting in her environment.

Babies with cerebral palsy frequently have squints (see below). The baby will have greater difficulty with visual attention and lose learning opportunities. Tracking an object may also be hampered by poor head control and persisting primary reflexes, and the immobile baby, or the baby with restricted movement, is prevented from exploring points of visual interest in her environment.

Children with hemiplegia may also have a hemianopia and ignore information from the affected side. Other more serious field defects occur and require careful evaluation (see section 7.2).

As in other types of learning, an inability to control what the baby looks at hampers the child's interaction with people and toys in her environment. Limited glimpses of the world and limited opportunities to experiment by implementing play schemata, lead not only to impoverished knowledge of the world, but also to poor motivation to explore it further. Visual attention is at risk if the child's ability to look at the dominant stimulus for any length of time is limited.

2.4.2 DEVELOPMENT OF VISUAL PERCEPTION

'The infant begins life with an impressive ability to make sense of her perceptions of people and things' (Bower, 1977). Bower goes on to quote many experiments showing that the newborn baby, to some extent, lives in a unified perceptual world with some degree of intersensory coordination. Researchers have shown that very young babies have some perception of emptiness, hardness, direction and distance. Babies are particularly responsive to face-like shapes, particularly those suggesting the presence of eyes. From 6 months onwards, with their hands fully operational in terms of reaching and grasping, they can experiment with toys and objects and learn more about their essential qualities.

By the end of the first year, the baby has learned to use distinctive features to identify an object represented pictorially and is able to perceive and predict essential characteristics in her environment.

(a)   Implications of physical handicap

Restricted movement limits or prevents interaction with the environment. First, the baby who cannot choose where she moves to has limited control over her visual input. Perceptual development is enhanced when the baby is able to be independently mobile in the exploration of the environment.

Bower (1977) quotes an experiment by Held, where two kittens are housed together, one being able to move while the other is held in a cradle. The visual input to both kittens is the same, but, on release, it was noted that the kitten who had not been active knew far less about its environment than the kitten who had been able to move. That babies with cerebral palsy may suffer similarly from their restricted movement has to be considered.

Secondly, the baby who has limited use of her hands will not glean as much information about the nature of her world as the baby who can grasp, pat, poke and stroke. If the hands are fisted or subject to a prolonged grasp reflex, the baby will not be able to use a flat hand to stroke or pat, thereby missing textural information. The baby with an indwelling thumb and hypertonic fingers will have difficulty opening the fingers but, even when she manages it, will find mouthing a toy and releasing it equally difficult. As a significant amount of information about the world comes to the baby via her mouth, her perceptual input is thereby restricted.

2.5   Play in the first year

Newborn babies have a broad repertoire of skills which enable them to begin to structure information from the environment. They can attend to visual and auditory stimuli, track objects, show pattern preference and complex manipulative exploration of the face and mouth. In their early months, babies, through social play, glean most of their information from people, particularly their mother. Social play then becomes the medium for the introduction of objects which the young baby will watch and track.

As experimentation with the movement of her own body progresses, the baby is likely to combine these movements with an interest in toys, and learns to grasp and mouth objects and subsequently to reach out for them. The baby may then build up a routine for investigating objects, for example, grasp, mouth, shake, mouth, regard, mouth, drop. At this stage, the baby's attention is easily diverted by novel stimuli. Exploratory play continues throughout the first year and is enhanced by the beginnings of symbolism, which is marked by the development of object permanence. From approximately 6 months, the baby is able to show her appreciation of certain routines and regularities in her life, and she will search for objects which have moved out of sight. As she approaches her first birthday the baby will show her level of symbolic understanding in her play, for example by pretending to drink from cup-like containers, brushing a doll's hair, trying to feed the dolly with her own dinner, etc. Around this time the baby's attention development allows her to include both people and objects in her play. The development of this concept of cause and effect, and her ability to anticipate events, allows the baby, at about 1 year, to initiate object play with an adult, and to pursue her own ideas in spite of the adult's attempts to vary the game.

2.5.1 IMPLICATIONS FOR CHILDREN WITH CEREBRAL PALSY

Play depends on social and physical interaction with the environment. Interaction with people and objects may be compromised by visual defect or by the visual sequelae of physical handicap. Poor head control may result in the baby missing the opportunity to associate visual and auditory stimuli. As the baby may not have the opportunity to develop body awareness, the degree of effort and experimentation to gain the same level of experience as a child without physical handicap is greater and may not be achievable in certain circumstances.

Abnormal patterns of movement may interfere with early play patterns, for example, if the child wishes to reach out to grasp a toy, this movement may produce involuntary movements in part of, or in the whole of, the baby's body. Her head may move so that visual contact with the toy is lost. Under these circumstances, the child will find first-hand investigation of the environment extremely difficult. Having little reward for her initiative, the baby may not sustain the effort to play. This may lead to frustration and apathy. Although the aspects of learning which rely on physical interaction with the environment are affected by physical impairment, not all cognitive areas are thus affected. Eagle (1985) was able to demonstrate that, in a sample of children with severe spastic quadriplegia, some children had developed a sophisticated level of the concept of object permanence without having had opportunities to be active in exploration, and concluded that, in this group of children, the development of object permanence was more dependent on *intellectual ability* than on motor skills. Impairment of motor function may mean, however, that the child is unable to pursue her own plans in play, and will be very reliant on the type of toys and the type of development of her playskills that adults choose for her.

2.5.2   PARENT AND PROFESSIONAL TASKS

(a)   Vision, perception, playing and learning

The parents' main task will be to provide the experiences the baby would normally gain from physical activity. This requires keen awareness of the baby's interest and accordingly much time and attention devoted to the baby. The parents need to know the nature of any visual or perceptual problems in order to modify their approaches to the child. They also need to interpret the infant's signals, both pre-intentional and intentional (e.g. limb movement, eye pointing). Interpreting such signals as meaningful may help to reinfore the baby's efforts to interact with people and objects.

The parents have to help the child to control her body so that her eyes can move without being restricted by reflex patterns and without all physical effort being expended on motor control. This will maximize visual and physical exploration. The primary need here is for a variety of stable play positions, if necessary using specially adapted seating or equipment (see Part Three). The equipment should be easily movable to different areas of the house, so that the baby has opportunities to experience different settings.

Various toys and common objects, e.g. wrist bells, coloured ribbons, cups, spoons, etc., can then be introduced, perhaps either attached to the baby herself, or hanging from a chair within reach of the baby. Once in a stable position, the baby can be encouraged to put her hands onto and into a variety of objects, so that she can learn the maximum information about shape, texture, hardness, etc.

If one side of the child's body only is affected, the affected hand should be included in play as much as possible. Some types of play will require considerable adult intervention (e.g. operating a toy). Encouraging the child to bear weight through her arms from as early an age as possible will also be helpful in enhancing proprioceptive awareness and in controlling abnormal tone.

Professionals need to encourage and reinforce parental skills in meeting the baby's needs. Part of this will be to provide advice on activities appropriate to the baby's developmental achievement and physical problems. Professionals should seek to develop parents' resources rather than provide specialized treatment which they cannot implement at home. Specific therapy and guidance is only one part of management, the overall aim of which is to foster parental independence and self-reliance. Achieving the balance between parental decision-making and professional activity requires considerable negotiation and tact, and will vary from time to time, and from family to family.

2.6 Care

Parents will expect a baby to be dependent in all aspects of everyday care. The baby with cerebral palsy, however, may be particularly difficult to care for, making considerable demands on her parents' time and skill. Difficulty or failure in meeting a baby's basic everyday needs can undermine parents' confidence in their parenting skills. Everyday care routines such as changing, bathing, feeding and dressing are also important contact times for parent and child. The availability of advice, support and aids from an early stage can help to promote more relaxed and positive contact between a parent and a child with cerebral palsy, and enable the parents to remain confident and in control of the care of their child.

2.6.1 EATING AND DRINKING

The normal development of eating and drinking involves the baby in learning to master an increasing range of oral movements with ever-finer control over an increasing variety of foods.

Suckling is the first feeding behaviour to occur. The baby needs to be able to find the nipple or teat as it touches her cheek or lips; to be able to make rapid transition from crying to suckling; to achieve a good oral seal with her lips; to cup the tongue effectively and to suckle with adequate strength to squirt the milk into the mouth. Babies are able to start and stop suckling easily and usually suckle with a rhythm of approximately one suck per second.

From about 3 months the baby may be introduced to solids, starting with bland baby rice and gradually increasing in taste and texture until, by the end of the first year, the baby may finger feed herself with a biscuit and eat a chopped up family meal. The introduction of solids has both sensory and motor implications.

The baby is highly adaptable at this stage, and progressively develops sensory tolerance to the variety of tastes, textures and temperatures to which she is introduced. A number of new oral movements are developed as the baby learns to tackle solids, such as closed mouth swallowing and lateral tongue and jaw movements. Towards the end of the first year the baby is given opportunities to drink from cups and thus develops strategies for dealing with liquids, progressing towards a mature swallowing pattern.

Mealtimes provide mother and baby with many social and emotional opportunities. The baby held in her mother's arms for breast or bottle feeding can make eye contact and learn to appreciate feeding rhythm. If the baby stops suckling momentarily, mother will look at her and perhaps jiggle her until suckling starts again. This soon establishes a turn-taking pattern. Behaviours such as eye avoidance, pulling away, cries or sound offer rich opportunities for the person feeding to interpret the baby's behaviour. Many babies learn to exert considerable control over their carers during feeding, and increased independence in feeding themselves is often a relief to mother and baby.

In addition, mealtimes, being highly motivating for the baby, help the child to develop an understanding and anticipation of events and language within a fairly consistent framework.

(a)   Implications of physical handicap

Tone abnormalities may disrupt the acquisition of normal feeding patterns, even mild fluctuations possibly resulting in poor coordination of suckling and swallowing.

(i) Suckling   The baby may find it difficult to initiate suckling and to maintain it if there is a poor oral seal, lack of stamina and no rhythm established. There may be difficulty in coordinating suckling, with swallowing resulting in gagging, aspiration and fear of feeding. A nasogastric tube may be introduced to provide adequate intake of food.

(ii) Solids   A baby with hypertonia may show jaw extension when her mouth is approached or touched by a spoon. This precludes her taking the food from the spoon with her top lip. The temptation to scrape the food off on her top teeth or gums may prove too great for the carer with the possible result that the food may drop onto the tongue and move down the pharynx to produce a gag reflex. Alternatively, the food may remain stuck to the hard palate. The baby's attempts to deal with solid food may be disrupted by persisting rooting and suckling reflexes, which may be stimulated by touch on the face or the palms of the hand. The resulting protrusion of the tongue means that the food is pushed out of the mouth. It may then be scraped off the chin by the

carer, triggering further reflex response. A vicious circle of feeding difficulty may result.

If a baby is slow to feed, impatience may result in larger and larger spoonsful of food being presented to the child. This may or may not include chin scraping; rapid feeding of large spoonsful will then result in even more food being pushed out of the mouth.

(iii) Drinking The baby may approach the drinking vessel with a suckle pattern. The up-and-down jaw movement in suckling will make liquids difficult to control both in the cup and in the mouth, with resulting dribbling and spillage and possibly choking.

(iv) Sensitivity The range of tastes and textures in food allows the baby to develop independence by offering opportunities for exploration within the situation. The baby with disordered sensation may react adversely to some tastes and textures. This may have the effect of discouraging the carer from introducing new tastes. Sensation difficulties are thus compounded as experiential possibilities are reduced.

The exploration of the properties of the food that comes with self-feeding towards the end of the first year is vital for learning about food. Self-feeding, or at least as much involvement with mealtime as possible, should be encouraged.

2.6.2 SOCIAL IMPLICATIONS

As the baby needs food for survival, feeding problems can cause much anxiety and distress in families. As parents find themselves unable to provide adequate nourishment for their baby, this causes fundamental feelings of inadequacy and extra time may be spent trying to feed the baby which will affect the life of the family. The baby may pick up tension and stress in the family, particularly in her mother, as well as the fundamental stress caused by discomfort during feeding and possibly a fear of choking. Children with this sort of difficulty may grow slowly as the primary result of their disorder, and slow weight gain increases anxiety.

Parents need considerable support during times of difficult feeding. A large part of this support will be advice and practical help in techniques to establish better feeding in the baby (see Chapter 11).

It may be some relief to the parents to find that their child is a difficult child to feed, and that the problem does not lie with them. Also, if the child is able to feed in the most efficient and therapeutic way, anxiety should be reduced to an extent. Reassurance about the amount of intake, could be offered by a dietitian, and an established routine at feeding time, will help to relieve the pressure on the rest of the family. Eating problems usually require short-term intensive bursts of therapy so that they can offer maximum support in establishing new feeding techniques and routines.

2.6.3 HANDLING

A normal baby can seem fragile and difficult to handle; the baby with cerebral palsy will be even more so. The baby will have a tendency to changes in tone and primitive reflexes, and many mothers find every-day activities of holding and carrying their child stressful.

In addition, these constantly repeated activities are a good opportunity to encourage and develop early gross motor skills and to use positions which inhibit abnormal reflex activity. At the same time, the infant can be held and carried in ways which encourage independent head control and enable her to look around and be aware of her environment.

Bathing a baby who has poor head control, very low tone, hyper-tonicity, or some involuntary movement, can be a difficult and frighten-ing experience for parents. For the small baby the use of a wedge in a baby bath can provide a safe, secure reclining position, keeping the head out of water and preventing involuntary movement. As the infant grows and needs a larger bath, a similar secure reclining position can be attained with the use of an aid in an adult bath. Parent's hands can be free for washing and the back strain caused by holding securely and washing at the same time can be prevented.

3 The early years

3.1 Family issues

3.1.1 LATER DIAGNOSIS

When a diagnosis of cerebral palsy is made outside the first year, it is likely to be of a milder or more specific form of the condition. Doctors and therapists may have a fairly optimistic view as to the child's potential to achieve good function and may be surprised by the degree of distress expressed by some parents when given the diagnosis. The severity of the handicapping condition is, of course, a major contributing factor to parental stress at diagnosis, but there are many other factors which will determine parents' perception of, reaction to and ability to cope with the diagnosis of cerebral palsy in their child.

(a) Prior awareness

The degree to which parents have been aware of their child's difficulties prior to diagnosis varies. A few with some awareness will have gone to considerable lengths to deny any problems by avoiding contact with doctors and health visitors. Others, particularly those with little experience of young children's development, may have remained unaware of the condition. Laborde and Seligman (1983) suggest that parents who have for some time perceived their child as normal, may have difficulty in acknowledging the disability. This will have implications for initiating therapy within the family.

Many parents, concerned and anxious about their child's development, may have experienced difficulty in getting doctors and others to recognize the problem, and may have been told to 'go away and stop worrying'. These parents may reasonably express anger towards doctors and health service professionals and there may be difficulties in establishing mutually trusting, therapeutic relationships.

(b) Attitudes to disability

Prior to the diagnosis, the majority of parents will have attitudes to disability that resemble those of the general public (Darling and

Darling, 1982). The label 'cerebral palsy' has been found to be perceived negatively by the general public, relative to other disabilities
(Barsch, 1964). Even those parents who are aware of a delay or specific
problem affecting a leg or an arm, may be distressed by the label
'cerebral palsy' and by the accompanying disclosure of long-term disability and of underlying brain damage.

(c)   Attachment

Parental response to the diagnosis of a disability in their infant's
second or third year will also be influenced by the quality of the
attachment relationship they have built up with their child in the
preceding months. This importance of the development of parent–
infant attachment in the first year is widely acknowledged as having
implications for the child's social and emotional development. Blacher
(1984) suggests that the quality of attachment between parent and
disabled child may influence family accord or discord, parents' ability
to collaborate with service providers, parent 'burnout', and even
eventual out-of-home placement. It has been suggested that, when
parents have formed an attachment to a child they see as 'normal',
they will find the disclosure of a disability particularly traumatic, and
will have difficulty accepting their child's disability (Lonsdale, 1978;
Blacher, 1984). These parents will need help and support in recognizing and adjusting to their child's disability before they can become
positively involved in his therapy.

It cannot be assumed, however, that because a diagnosis was not
made until later, the early parent–infant attachment will have pro-
ceeded normally. Attachment formation between parent and infant
requires both partners to be active and interactive. A child with cerebral palsy may give attenuated cues to the parents and may be slow in
responding. The parents may be unsure in handling him and lacking in
confidence, and may well report that they 'felt that something was
wrong from the day he was born'. These parents may find acceptance
of the eventual diagnosis less difficult, but will have particular needs
for therapeutic intervention which will foster the development of
warmth and reciprocity between parent and child, facilitate mutual
understanding and communication, and enhance parental confidence.

Whether the diagnosis is made at birth or much later, parents must
be viewed as having particular needs in the period after diagnosis.
They will need time to assimilate the information, and opportunity to
talk with professionals and others about the diagnosis and its implications for their child and family. In this way they begin gradually to
construct an understanding for themselves. Barsch (1968) points out
that parents whose child's disability is recognized later in his develop-

ment face the special challenge of undergoing gradual changes in their thinking about the child at the same time as coping with rapid changes in the child's life.

3.1.2 ADJUSTMENT

Even those families who have accepted the diagnosis of disability in their child and who have had access to good information, counselling and support around the time of diagnosis, continue to experience increasing levels of stress as the child grows up. This appears not to relate simply to age, but to significant events or transformations in the family's life cycle (Wikler *et al.*, 1981). Blacher (1984) suggests that it is more helpful to view parental adjustment as fluid so that, rather than reaching one final level of acceptance, parents experience periods of acceptance throughout the life of their child. The toddler period is one in which significant changes occur in the transition from baby to child, and many new challenges and stresses are presented to parents of infants with cerebral palsy.

Perhaps of greatest significance is the change in expectations of and demands on the infant. Toddlers and young children must walk and talk, and the failure of the infant with cerebral palsy to master these skills makes his disability much more visible, both to his parents and to their network of family/friends and acquaintances.

A physical disability in a baby may have caused no disruption to the routines of family life, and at this stage it is relatively easy to maintain beliefs that the disability is minimal, temporary, or perhaps subject to 'cure' by physiotherapy. The realities of the child's development in the toddler period are likely to challenge this. As the child struggles to master motor skills, his disability may appear to worsen. The physical effort will increase his muscle tone and this hypertonicity will make him appear much more abnormal than he was as a 'floppy' baby.

Parents may also have to cope with emerging evidence of additional disabilities. Many children with cerebral palsy are likely to have some degree of associated learning difficulty and it is during the second, third and fourth years that significant delays in cognitive development will become apparent. Intellectual ability is highly valued in our culture, and some parents will find adjustment to a mental handicap more difficult than their acceptance of their child's motor disability. As the child faces the challenges of the toddler period, more specific difficulties with language and communication skills may also be identified. Parents who had rebuilt their hopes and expectations for their child around positive development in areas where they believed his physical disability would not affect him, may suffer repeated disappointments as these new problems emerge.

During this period, parents may also have to adjust to the intrusions of professionals into areas of child care and development which would normally be their sole responsibility. The rapid changes and developments of this age make appropriate intervention and therapy particularly crucial if the child's progress is to be optimal, and the use of maladaptive movement patterns is to be prevented. Most parents will have no previous experience of dealing with professionals and will find this an additional stress.

It is essential that service providers balance the child's needs for intervention and therapy with parental requirements for counselling, support and time to reflect and make an adjustment.

3.1.3   WORKING WITH FAMILIES

There will be individual differences in the way families organize themselves in order to cope on a day-to-day basis with meeting the needs of a child with a disability. The balance of relationships and the degree of openness of communication and cooperation existing in families prior to the birth of a child with a disability will influence their ability to cope emotionally and physically.

The involvement of parents in, and their commitment to, therapeutic intervention is particularly crucial for a toddler with cerebral palsy. Relative to parents of children with developmental delays and mental handicaps, the parents of children with cerebral palsy will need to learn much more specialized techniques for handling, positioning, teaching and facilitating their child's development.

(a)   Parental roles

In most two-parent families, fathers and mothers have distinct and different roles with regard to child-rearing. Individual families define roles according to their own choices and needs, and in many families now, traditional roles may be merged or reversed. Nevertheless, in a large proportion of families, day-to-day childcare may still be seen as women's work. Where a child has cerebral palsy, it will tend to be the mother, during the child's early years, who attends therapy or is at home when therapists call. She is also the one who meets other mothers of children with disabilities, who carries out the therapy and teaching with her child, and who questions and talks with professionals on a day-to-day basis. In a large number of families, therefore, it is only the mothers who have the degree of access to experiences which will enable them to develop a realistic knowledge of their child's disability, and which will enable them to make a greater adjustment. In families with less than optimal communication, the gap between the mother's and the father's knowledge and adjustment may continue to widen. Lamb (1983) suggests that this can lead to significant stresses and more serious problems in the family. Services initially child-focused are now increasingly mother–child focused, but it is clearly important to seek and maintain the involvement of both parents so that fathers not involved in day-to-day care are able to share in the knowledge and awareness of the child's problems and participate actively in goal planning and problem solving.

(b) Siblings

During the early years, siblings will experience the disruption of family routines caused by frequent hospital trips and numerous home visits, where attention is focused on their younger sibling. The impact of a child with a disability is not necessarily negative in the longer term for his siblings, who may encounter unusual opportunities for growth and development. Nevertheless, stress in the family will pose risks to their social and emotional development, and inter-family relationships may be affected. Where a child requires a high degree of physical care, siblings may be given responsibilities in excess of those usually given to children of their age. They may also have anxieties about 'catching' the disability, or fear they themselves may be in some way defective. These problems may be particularly acute in the case of twins and higher order births, where the incidence of cerebral palsy is higher.

The most significant determinant of a child's ability to adopt a positive attitude to, and cope with, his younger brother or sister's disability will be his parents' attitude and adjustment. This in turn will be influenced by the information, counselling and support that they themselves have received from professional services during the toddler stage. Parents tend to become very involved in organizing for the child with cerebral palsy, and it may be up to the professional to direct attention to the needs and problems of the siblings. Parents need to be enabled to communicate the nature of a child's handicap at a level and in terms which the other children in the family can understand.

(c) Professional roles

Successful negotiation of therapeutic involvement is the professionals' task. A failure on the part of professionals to engage parents in therapy will not only lead to a lack of developmental progress, but also to a deterioration in longer-term function as the child continues to use maladaptive postures and movement patterns.

Parents and professionals need to have a clear understanding of each other's viewpoints. They must be able to communicate openly and negotiate mutual therapeutic commitment, based on the professional's specialist assessment of the child's needs, and on an understanding of the parents' views, aims, expectations, current situation and resources. Failure to resolve differences in parent and professional expectations at this point is likely to render therapeutic input ineffective. In the absence of good communication and clear negotiation, some parents may respond by handing over responsibility to the experts, while others may avoid contact with professionals or more simply ignore advice and recommendations.

Individual workers, whatever their professional background, will become involved in counselling and supporting parents. They in turn will need opportunities to develop these skills, and access to support systems to allow them to undertake these tasks within a family.

Where more than one person is involved with a child with cerebral palsy, the potential for parental confusion over conflicting goals and approaches to the child is very high. For example, the physiotherapist may use a toy to encourage a child to maintain sitting balance while using his hands in play, whereas the teacher brings the same toy and suggests that the parents use a corner seat so that he can concentrate on play with his hands. To parents, they seem to be doing the same. In addition to good communication between individual professionals and parents, it is also vital that professionals have good communication among themselves and a system of coordination. A team of professionals should include parents in all its discussions relevant to the child. One of the team may be given the role of key worker, and act as the main link between the team and the parents.

While there is general acceptance of the benefit of enabling parents to teach and carry out therapy programmes with their child, there are notable pitfalls to these approaches. Parents who become successful teachers or therapists may do so at the cost of becoming less of a parent (Wright, 1982). Following parent training programmes, parents may view themselves more as teacher than parent (Baker, 1980) and experience additional pressures to 'do well'. The parent's feeling of being evaluated can create yet another source of stress affecting interaction with the child (Wright, 1982) and significantly change the sources of enjoyment which parents gain from their child, so that they focus on progress and successes rather than on more everyday pleasures, such as enjoying the child's company (Jones, 1980). Kogan *et al.* (1974) compared mother–child interactions of children with cerebral palsy while mother and child played together and while they engaged in performing therapy. During therapy the mother and child showed greater amounts of negative behaviour (e.g. control, hostility, intrusion, ambiguous affect, negative voice and content) than when they were playing. These differences persisted over a two-year period, and over this period the positive interactions during play sessions declined.

Parents have a variety of interacting styles (Bromvich, 1976). Professionals should be sensitive to individual family styles and choices and aware of the impact of involvement in therapy and teaching on the parent–child relationship. Therapeutic approaches can then be tailored to individual family needs. Physiotherapy will almost inevitably involve 'hands on' work with the child, but the extent to which the therapist interacts with the child during sessions and models for the parent, or allows the parent to handle the child while giving guidance and feedback, can be varied to suit individual families. Where intervention is focused on language, social or cognitive development, it may be possible to conduct sessions using observation, commentary and discussion, rather than training and modelling approaches.

Enabling both parent and child to enjoy therapy and teaching sessions will go far in preventing the more negative effects of intervention on the parent–child relationship. The integration of therapy into everyday activities will also help to maintain parents in their essential parenting role.

3.1.4 SOCIAL SUPPORT

In most families, the everyday stresses of having a lively young child are alleviated by social support. This may consist of extended informal networks of family, friends, neighbours and fellow-parents, or of more formal resources such as the health visitor, mother and toddler groups and toy libraries. Social networks are sources of information, advice, practical and emotional support and, at times, respite.

Parents whose child has a significant disability such as cerebral palsy tend to make less use of social support networks. There are practical reasons for this, in that it may be easier for them to seek advice and support in everyday child-rearing and health care issues from the specialist professionals involved with the child, and they may have little opportunity to make neighbourhood contacts, and no time to attend local mother and toddler groups. Moreover, it is likely that a parent whose child is visibly disabled finds talking to others about the child stressful, and limiting contact to close family and specialist professionals minimizes this stress (Waisbren, 1980; Wright *et al.*, 1984). In the longer term, however, there is evidence that parenting of a child with a disability is less stressful if there is good social support. The size of the social network is less important than the perception by parents of the quality of this support.

It is clearly important that professionals working with the child and family have an awareness of the risks of isolating parents from local social networks, and of the consequences of this, both for the parents' long-term coping ability and the social integration of the child within his neighbourhood. One of the goals of services should be to facilitate the parent and child's functioning as part of their neighbourhood network.

Parents may need specific counselling and support to enable them to make new contacts or renew old ones, to talk about their child and his disability, participate in mother and toddler groups, and interact with other parents in playgroups or nurseries. They will also need help in coping with negative reactions and experiences of rejection. Some parents, although by no means all, value contact with others of similarly disabled children. These groups reduce isolation and, although not directly facilitating neighbourhood contacts, may be useful in giving parents confidence to make contacts outside their 'disability network'.

3.1.5 NURSERY AND PLAYGROUP

At some point the parent of a child with cerebral palsy will be asked to consider whether they wish to send their child to a nursery or preschool playgroup. These settings are generally regarded as helping a child to develop social competence and enabling him to cope with the school-type routines, as well as giving valuable learning opportunities and independence. Nursery may also provide much needed respite for parents.

As the child with cerebral palsy may require specialized physical care, some parents may not feel that the local nursery staff are competent in handling their child. They may be protective and reluctant to trust other adults with his care or expose their child and themselves to possible rejection and insensitive reactions from other members of the public. They know also that their child who is able to be mobile in his own home will be physically at risk from contact with more physically able and energetic peers. However, although placing a child in a special nursery with others with similar special needs has obvious advantages, such as concentrated expert handling and appropriate materials, the parents may worry that the opportunity to interact with able-bodied children with a certain level of communicative competence may be lost.

Integrating the child with cerebral palsy into his local nursery may seem desirable socially, but will need careful thought and possibly increased manpower if the child is to participate fully in nursery life. Making choices and decisions about nursery placement can be difficult for parents, who may face rejection of their child by nurseries which feel they cannot cope with the child's special needs.

When the child attends an integrated nursery, the parents may experience stress on seeing their child's disability in the context of his non-disabled peers. Around the time of nursery placement, the parents will need clear information and support. They must be given opportunities to express their fears and anxieties and discuss their feelings. They will need concrete information on the level of care that will be available to their child, and will need to make visits to various resources without feeling pressure to accept one.

Once in the nursery the child will need some professional support from therapists, support teachers, etc., but nursery should not be seen as the primary location of care. In his early years, the parents continue to be the most important resource for the child. They should continue to be closely involved in the child's therapy. Many parents have a considerable degree of expertise in the management of their child and should be considered part of the team.

3.2   Interacting

3.2.1   SOCIALIZATION

The second year of life sees the onset of socialization pressure. The infant is expected to take his first steps into the wider social world and to acquire the knowledge and skills which will enable him to function with some independence of his parents, and yet behave in a way which reflects their values and those of the social group to which they belong.

Between his second and fifth year, the child develops the ability to interpret his own and others' feelings and to express emotions appropriately. He begins to monitor and control his own behaviour, becoming less dependent on immediate parental controls. His play with peers becomes increasingly interactive and cooperative and he makes his first friends. By 5 years of age the child's social maturity should enable him to cope with the demands of school life.

In his early years the child's social and emotional development is, to some extent, facilitated by his development in other areas. Physical development allows him to be more mobile and less dependent on adult help; cognitive development, in particular the emergence of representational thinking, enables the child to use thought to understand his social world. His behaviour can be based on recollections of past events and prediction of likely consequences. Communication skills also develop rapidly during this period. In the second year, even before the emergence of verbal language, the infant becomes a more insistent, specific and effective communicator, and there is a change from proximal to distal modes of communication between parent and child. As language skills develop, verbal communication assumes an increasingly important role in the child's social relationship.

For the child with cerebral palsy, social and emotional development may not proceed smoothly. His physical handicap will hinder his independence, communication skills may be impaired, and for some children there will be the additional challenge of intellectual impairment. In addition, a child with a disability such as cerebral palsy may well have had difficulties in establishing good quality early attachment relationships (Blacher and Meyers, 1983), which are, in turn, related to subsequent competence and confidence in separation, peer relationships, communication skills and self-control (Ainsworth and Bell, 1974; Matas *et al.*, 1978).

Interventions designed to enhance the child's functioning in other areas of his development may hinder his social and emotional development. One example of this may be seen in the negative effects of very controlling and directive parenting on the development of self-control. Young children with cerebral palsy are likely to experience much more parental control and direction, particularly in the implementation of therapy programmes but also in the course of their day-to-day life, than is usual at this age. The child's therapeutic programme may also dominate his life to the extent that there is little time or opportunity to be separate from a carer, play casually alongside peers and observe and try out new social skills. Some children may spend their early years largely in the company of adults or that of children with similar disabilities. Their opportunities for establishing peer friendships with socially interactive peers and for modelling socially competent and appropriate behaviours may be severely affected.

There is plentiful evidence that children with physical disabilities experience a higher than average level of social and emotional difficulties, and that children whose disability is associated with a neurological impairment are particularly at risk of socio-emotional disorders (McMichael, 1971; Seidel *et al.*, 1975; Anderson, *et al.*, 1982). While intellectual factors do influence social and emotional development and there is an association between low intelligence and socio-emotional difficulties, intellectual factors do not account in total for the discrepancy in rates of psychiatric difficulty between children whose physical handicap is and is not associated with underlying brain damage. When comparisons are made between groups of children of average intelligence, the children with neurologically based physical disabilities have higher rates of psychiatric difficulty than children whose physical handicaps are not associated with underlying brain damage (Rutter *et al.*, 1970).

(a)   Intervention

Social and emotional development may not appear to be a priority for the child with cerebral palsy in the early years. This is likely to be as a result of intensive work on more visible areas of his development, such as speech and mobility. Social and emotional difficulties are also less evident in the young child, coming to prominence in later childhood and adolescence. Wasserman *et al.* (1985), however, report observations of a higher rate of behaviours such as passivity, inhibition, reluctance to separate, distractibility and low compliance in children with physical handicaps as young as 2 years, when compared with their non-disabled peers. Many professionals who work with young children with disabilities would confirm this finding. The toddler and preschool period can be very stormy for some children with cerebral palsy, who may be exceptionally clingy to their parent, show extreme distress on separation or be unable to cope with the pressures of therapy, responding with frequent tantrums or withdrawal.

Any goal planning and strategy selection during the child's early years should focus positively on the tasks of social and emotional development, and the child's social and emotional needs should be acknowledged in planning for other areas of his skill development. This can be achieved by interdisciplinary teamwork where the parent is a full member of the team. The team should be able to use their knowledge of the child and his strengths and difficulties, together with their knowledge of socio-emotional development of this childhood period, to ensure that his development in this, as in other areas, is optimal, and to prevent as far as possible later socio-emotional difficulty.

The major socialization tasks of the early years are as follows.

(i) Developing effective communication   While reciprocal smiling and vocalization might be appropriate for babies, in the second year infants should be developing much more specific and insistent communication. Parents may need to be discouraged from anticipating needs and encouraged to watch for, and respond to, communicative signals such as eye pointing, hand pointing and specific vocalizations. The child must learn to make demands and choices, before he can progress to

words, signs or a picture/symbol system. He needs to learn that he can influence his social environment and be effective within it.

(ii) Separation   As far as possible, the child with a physical disability should be given the same degree of control over initial separations as his non-disabled peer. This may be achieved by giving some form of independent mobility in the home, allowing him to follow his parent and initiate separations and reunions. When he is not mobile, he should be able to see his parent, or be reassured by voice, and his parent should be encouraged to respond to his signals for reunion. The infant will also need some play activities at which he is competent without parental help and support. Where a child also has an intellectual impairment, he may need more time and learning opportunities in order to separate happily from his carer, and he may, therefore, continue to need the reassurance of his carer's presence when he is chronologically old enough for nursery. A gradual introduction to the nursery with his parent and a handover to a key worker who can give close and consistent attention should enable the child to make a smooth transition and avoid distress when he is left at nursery. Many parents will also need considerable support when loosening their ties with a child who has been so dependent on them, consumed so much of their time and seems frail and vulnerable alone in his nursery or playgroup.

(iii) Playing with peers and making friends   The toddler with a physical disability may be overwhelmed by a mother and toddler group, with a lot of mobile toddlers, and will be able to make few social contacts in this setting. However, his peer social skills will be facilitated by regular meetings, preferably in his own home, with one or two other children. At some stage attendance at a nursery or playgroup may be beneficial, allowing the child to acquire and practise social skills in a more challenging setting. Where possible the child should be enabled to continue in his relationships with neighbourhood children prior to going to school. Some children, particularly those with very severe disabilities, may not be able to attend their neighbourhood nursery. All nurseries should, however, be able to offer a child opportunities for peer group interaction and social learning. Successful integration of a child into a nursery will require the adults to play an active part in ensuring his full participation in the social activities of the nursery.

(iv) Self-control   Is it possible to learn to be good without opportunities to be naughty? Close directive, restrictive or protective parenting limits the child's learning through his self-initiated actions. He needs time which is not directed, and opportunities to participate in the same

range of social situations as non-disabled toddlers. Family mealtimes, for example, can be an important exercise for learning social rules from which the child with feeding difficulties may be excluded. Parents may also need to be encouraged to apply the same rules to the disabled child's behaviour as they would to other children in the family, when the child's physical and communicative competences are taken into account.

3.2.2 COMMUNICATION IN THE EARLY YEARS

While language continues to develop into adolescence, it is during the early years that the most dramatic developments occur. Although the baby learns to communicate efficiently, it is as a toddler that he is expected to become linguistically capable. Through play with adults and objects, the child learns social and cognitive boundaries. By experimenting with using single words, the child learns semantic boundaries, both receptively and expressively until, by approximately 18 months, the toddler may have a sizeable vocabulary. Two word utterance may begin to appear at this stage and at around 2 years short sentences may be used and understood. After a period where key words only are uttered, e.g. 'Mummy gone work car', grammatical features, such as plural and tense markers, are acquired gradually.

During the early years the child's language becomes increasingly important in the development of the concept of self, and the development of relationships with adults and other children outside the family. Language is required in important social situations such as parties and nursery interactions.

While the child's early uses of language are mainly for fulfilling his own needs and regulating the behaviour of others (Halliday, 1975), during the early years the child learns to use language to give and request information, express feelings and facilitate social contact. He also uses language during imaginative play.

The child's phonology and articulatory systems should also be maturing during this period, and by the fourth year, most parents expect intelligible speech.

There are many ways that language development can be compromised in the event of physical handicap. Severely delayed gross motor skills may compromise the child's ability to build up knowledge of the world through play and interaction. More control over the environment and the inability to try out new words to examine their semantic boundaries will affect the child's abilities to acquire language for use in communication. The use of expressive language enhances the development of comprehension (Clarke, 1974) which may equally be affected by the child's reduced ability to manifest his understanding.

This may lower people's expectations of the child, with the result that he is not stretched linguistically.

If the degree of motor disability is mild or moderate, the child may have some difficulty in developing a range of movements required for speech. Attempts to achieve precise articulatory movement may trigger unwanted patterns of movement, and there may be difficulty in coordinating breath and voice and subsequently tongue and jaw movement. These slowed mouth movements may result in slurred speech which may, at best, be difficult for the child's peers to understand and, at worst, cause teachers and others in the child's environment to interpret poor output and timing as a sign of intellectual impairment. Failure in spoken communication may be one of the child's early experiences as first attempts may be unintelligible. As a result of this, many children may be reluctant to talk in class or in groups and may find that they cannot join in with 'chats' because of poor timing.

Children who are severely affected by their physical disability may not be able to use oral communication to an effective extent. Many young children with cerebral palsy may well be able to make their needs known, although by means usually interpretable only by close family. Therefore, the introduction of a more conventional symbolic communication system is vital in the early stages to produce a need in the child to communicate specific ideas. If the system is introduced too late, the child will be reluctant to abandon his gross but efficient attempts at communication for a system which is essentially much more difficult if ultimately more accurate. Early introduction is also advisable to reduce the experience of failure and to increase motivation. A discussion of the advantages and disadvantages of an alternative system of communication can be found in Chapter 13.

For children needing oral communication, this may be a difficult period. The professionals may be able to advise on optimum position for breath control, pitch control and developing sound sequences, and help the child to develop the strategies to ensure efficient communication in spite of these difficulties to limit frustration. In our experience, however, children of this age have a poor motivation level for maximizing their physical potential orally, and formal speech therapy may have to be postponed until the child has a greater emotional maturity. Again technology may help here in interesting the child in otherwise possibly boring activities.

3.3   Independence in everyday care

Young children remain dependent on their parents for all aspects of their day-to-day care, but as they develop more skilled movements and their understanding and problem solving abilities increase, they participate more actively and effectively in the day-to-day routines of eating, drinking, dressing, bathing and using the potty. By the end of the fifth year the role of the parents in these activities will have changed from one of doing everything for the child to one of supervising and giving help and guidance where necessary.

Independence in self-care, or the ability to look after oneself, is highly valued in our culture. The schoolchild who cannot manage his clothes may well be teased by his peers, and even occasional incontinence in an older child can be a source of significant distress and embarrassment to parent and child. For children with disabilities considerable effort will be invested in working towards goals of autonomy and independence throughout their childhood and for some this will continue into their adult lives. For very young children, however, there is a degree of ambivalence towards the notion of the infant's decreasing dependence on his parents. Many parents and other adults are reluctant to lose the closeness of caring for the highly dependent baby. The desire to continue 'babying' the child in his second year is quite common, but the average toddler soon asserts his desire for autonomy. Donaldson (1978) argues that there is a fundamental urge to be effective, competent and independent, which is evident even in the young baby who shows signs of wanting to control his environment even at a stage when he is relatively helpless. This does not appear to derive from any rewards other than the achievement of competence and control. Papousek (1969), in his work on infant learning, was able to show that not only do infants not need a primary reward such as food for successful learning, but that they will behave in a way that produces results in the world for no reward other than that of a successful outcome and an accompanying sense of mastery. It may be assumed, therefore, that the child whose helplessness is the result of a physical disability still has a fundamental urge to have control over his environment, and enabling him to achieve this must be an important part of therapeutic intervention.

The infant who is not disabled will initiate and his parents will easily discern his readiness to undertake new learning and face new challenges. Such cues may be less readily available from the child with cerebral palsy, obscured not only by the child's motor handicap, which will make it much more difficult for parents to assess his motor potential for achieving any goal, but also by the possible disruption to the parent–infant relationship, which could cause parents to be less tuned in to their infant's responses and less able to reflect his choices and preferences. Very young children need to focus all their attention on the task involved. They can cooperate to some extent with adults if the adult's involvement is facilitative and enabling rather than intrusive and directive. The immediate goals of any action must be the child's rather than the adult's. Where attempts to establish independence are intrusive and adult-led, they will result in distress and resistance. There is also evidence that very young children have an awareness of their own success or failure in tasks; this is the first stage in the construction of their self-image. They will subsequently discover the value that others put upon them, and the views of adults and peers will be of increasing importance. These views in turn will be influenced by the child's apparent competence so that success in mastery of independence skills will have an impact both on the child's current self-image and on his future self-esteem.

Avoidance and withdrawal are quite natural responses to situations in which an individual cannot meet the challenges he has set for himself or which have been set for him by others. Bruner (1966) refers to this as coping versus defending, and there are individual differences as to the extent that children or adults will persevere in the teeth of failure. The child with cerebral palsy is likely to encounter failure even in working towards goals of his own choosing as well as being unable to meet the challenges set for him by others.

Working towards the development of independence skills in the infant with cerebral palsy is clearly a minefield. On the one hand there is a strong urge towards achievement and autonomy and the importance of mastery to the child's self-image and his future self-esteem; on the other hand there are the extreme difficulties faced by a child with a motor disorder in achieving success in these very motor-dependent skills. The risks of over-challenging the child and causing failure avoidance and a breakdown in the parent–child relationship co-exist with the risks of underachievement and possible long-term passivity and dependence. Some parents read their child easily and can generalize from his gross and fine motor abilities to his potential in self-help skills. They will need only access to aids and a little advice. Other parents will need much more help in ascertaining their child's readiness to progress to new areas of independence and will need guidance in adopting facilitative failure-free approaches.

3.3.1 EATING AND DRINKING

Eating and drinking have important social as well as nutritional functions. During the toddler stage the infant acquires the necessary sophistication to use a spoon without undue spillage, and to progress to a fork. His oral skills improve so that he develops rotary chewing with closed lips, and drinks from a cup without spillage. As hand and mouth coordinate more effectively, the toddler can give his attention to joining in social interactions and learning the social rules. By the end of his third year, a child will be able to participate in family mealtimes with minimal supervision of his eating and drinking skills.

At mealtimes the young child will indulge in messy play with food and utensils, through which he will learn much about the nature of food, independence in control and the limits of his parents' tolerance. Although the toddler can cope physically with most foods, he is much more aware of different tastes and textures, and is beginning to express his likes and dislikes quite strongly. Food fads and food refusal are common at this stage. Palmer *et al.* (1975) found, in a survery of behaviour problems in 3-year-olds, that 11% of the children had food fads.

Some children with cerebral palsy will not develop independence in self-feeding during the toddler period. This may be due to severity of motor disability affecting the upper limbs, or to more specific oral difficulties necessitating continued feeding intervention to improve oral function.

Parents of children with cerebral palsy may initially be reluctant to progress towards the independence of their child in feeding, because of anxieties about adequate nutritional intake. Although this may well have been a priority concern in the baby period, it is likely to be less of a problem in the young child because nutritional needs at this age do not increase at the same rate as those of the baby. Parents may need considerable reassurance about the adequacy of the child's nutritional intake before handing over control to a typically fussy and messy toddler, who will seem to put more food on his face and on the floor than in his mouth.

The child himself may not find the transition to self-feeding easy. If there have been early feeding difficulties, he may well have had mainly negative experiences of food and eating. If he is to master a skill which is much more difficult for him than for his non-disabled peer, he will need both the intrinsic enjoyment of food and a good rapport with his parent at mealtimes, to maintain his motivation.

Where the child tends to remain as part of a rather intense dyad, perpetuated from the baby years, with the focus of attention on him and his eating, and with very limited opportunities to assert his own control over food consumption, both infant and parent may, for different reasons, find the prolongation of feeding uncomfortable or stressful.

(a) Facilitating eating (see Chapter 9)

Feeding intervention at this stage must recognize the needs of toddler and family as different from those of parent and baby. Seating must provide, as for the baby, an optimal position for trunk and head and mouth control in feeding, but should also allow for some social participation in the family mealtimes. Although some families will find feeding more relaxed and pleasant when it is done in the course of their mealtimes, where the child's oral dysfunction is severe, requiring the complete involvement of one adult, feeding may continue to be separate.

Parents may find it helpful, at this stage, to involve other adults, such as grandparents, in feeding the child. This will lessen the intense parent–child interaction of feeding, allow for some respite, and give the toddler access to age-appropriate social opportunities of eating with friends or extended family. Parents may themselves be able to pass on expertise and techniques, but may also enlist the direct help of the therapist in teaching and giving confidence to new feeders.

Spoon-feeding involves fine motor manipulation, tool use, hand-to-mouth coordination and oral skills. Earlier experiences of object play (finger- and spoon-feeding, or holding a bottle or feeder cup during feeding) will all contribute to the child's acquisition of cup and spoon use. As with any activity using hand skills, careful attention will be required to ensure postural stability. Parents may need advice on adapting seating for mealtimes, or a special seat which will allow the child to sit at the family meal table. Spoon-feeding requires the skilled use of one hand, the other being positioned on the table in midline and holding the dish if appropriate, to give a stable position and avoid associated reactions.

(b)   Drinking

Young children are expected to make the change from breast feeding/bottle feeding to independent drinking from a cup. Children usually start with a feeder cup, i.e. a cup with a spout on the lid, to give independence while avoiding undue spillage. In the child with cerebral palsy, however, this type of nozzle may produce an unwanted suckling reflex, and parents may be advised to encourage the child to drink from a cut-out or slanted (Doidy) cup which, because of its shape, helps to inhibit such reflexes. In doing this, however, the parents will have to sacrifice a certain amount to their child's independence. It is important to help the parents achieve a balance between independence and good drinking patterns.

Extended dependency in eating should not necessarily deprive the young child of opportunities to sample, develop and express preferences for new tastes and textures, and therapy regimes should be geared towards expanding tolerance of a range of these. This is important in maintaining the infant's interest in what will at times be a tedious process. Finding ways of enabling the child to make active choices of food and drink, rather than waiting for him to refuse and reject what is offered, gives him some of the choices appropriate to the toddler stage.

Perhaps of most importance in this period is negotiation between the therapist and parents, so that a balance can be achieved between the child's needs for autonomy, the parents' desire for a relaxation of stressful feeding times, the need to develop good patterns, and the child's nutritional needs.

3.3.2 DEVELOPING CONTINENCE

Even the most superficial observation indicates that in our culture considerable emphasis is placed on the desirability of early toilet training. In a survey of infant care practices in Nottingham (Newson and Newson, 1976), 83% of mothers started toilet training before the age of 12 months (63% before 8 months). The parents surveyed were aware that continence by one year was unlikely, and of the possible negative effects of pressure on the baby, but were, Newsome concludes, so influenced by the subtle prestige attached to early and successful toilet training, that they would gamble that their child would be different. Some parents are, of course, very relaxed about toilet training, but there is an expectation that the toddler will achieve continence, though perhaps not total independence. However, the pressure on parents to train their child is increased when attendance at a preschool playgroup or nursery is a goal, as these resources usually require a child to be fairly independent as regards continence at as young as 3 years. For children with a physical disability, an opportunity to attend a local nursery or playgroup is an important first step towards successful integration with his local peer group, and toilet training can become a priority task in the early years.

The child has many skills, both physical and social, to acquire before he can be regarded as reliably continent. He must have acquired neurological maturity so that reflex systems can come under his voluntary control. Parents are often alert to these signs of 'readiness'. They notice changes in movement and body posture which indicate that the child is beginning to inhibit or 'hold on' and they are able to introduce the potty and have a reasonable chance of success. The child also needs to learn to inhibit and initiate urination and defecation involving voluntary coordination of the muscles of the pelvic floor, abdomen and diaphragm. He must learn what potties and toilets are, and that, though they may appear different from each other, they all have the same function. Initially his motivation to use his potty may come from parental feedback, but he will soon develop an awareness of the social implications of incontinence and will be upset by 'accidents' which are an inevitable part of the learning process.

The major problem for the child with cerebral palsy is likely to be in postural control and in control and coordination of the voluntary muscles involved. Parents may need advice about the right time to begin training. Unlike most young children, the child with a movement disorder may not give visible cues that he is inhibiting or initiating urination or defecation. Parents will find it more difficult to begin potty training by 'catching' the child and will perhaps need to talk to professionals about whether their child is developmentally ready for training to begin.

The young child with cerebral palsy is likely to need some form of additional support when using his potty (see Part 3). This may be in the form of a design of potty with good back and front support, or may involve the use of a special 'potty chair'. When sitting on the potty, the child should not be struggling to maintain postural stability and should feel safe, secure and relaxed. When special equipment is used, it will be important for parents and professionals to review the child's needs so that more ordinary potties can be substituted when appropriate.

Establishing faecal continence in a child with cerebral palsy may be complicated by constipation. Where eating and drinking have been difficult, poor diet and restricted fluid intake may cause problems. Even before potty training begins, the child's poor muscle tone, postural control and mobility may have inhibited natural defecation. If parents and professionals are aware of these hazards from an early age, appropriate steps on diet, handling and treatment can be taken before potty training, so that discomfort, pain and fear do not disrupt the child's learning of continence skills.

Once the child has the physical skills and is happy about using the potty, he progresses by indicating his needs non-verbally or verbally. Some children with cerebral palsy may well have difficulties in communicating, and help from professionals may be required either to enable parents to interpret the child's existing communication or to establish a way in which the child can signal his need. For children with less severe disabilities, toilet training may be straightforward until the point at which a greater degree of autonomy is required. The difficulties may then be in the child's ability to get to or onto a toilet without assistance and to manage his clothing. Some specific teaching may be necessary to enable the child to circumvent his physical difficulty and some simple adaptation in clothing may allow the degree of independence appropriate to his age level.

A proportion of children with cerebral palsy will not show age-appropriate independence in continence skills by the time they begin nursery. For these children it is important that appropriate adaptations and practical assistance are made available to them, and there is continuity of training from home to nursery.

3.3.3 DRESSING AND UNDRESSING

Although most young children will develop competence in undressing and acquire some independence in dressing, these skills do not, at this stage, have the same degree of social and cultural importance as self-feeding and toilet training. Parents tend not to organize themselves specifically to teach dressing skills, but will allow and encourage independence to emerge gradually.

For the child with severe motor impairment, dressing and undressing sessions may become more difficult and distressing as he grows bigger and becomes more active. The effort a child makes, whether intended to assist or (more typical of the very young child) to resist, during dressing is likely to result in increased tone (extension), and will make taking off and putting on clothes virtually impossible. Dressing and undressing sessions which have to occur several times daily may become increasingly unpleasant for those involved, and a major source of conflict between parent and child. For children with severe degrees of hypertonicity, establishing independence will not be an immediate goal of intervention in the early years. The priority will be to establish dressing as a relaxed and social time, where the child can learn about his body and perhaps have some active participation in the process. Advice on holding and positioning the child is crucial. Parents will need to position him so that hypertonicity is minimal and movements either active or passive can be facilitated. The use of body part rhymes and games, e.g. 'This little piggy', as part of the dressing routine will help both parties to relax and enhance the child's awareness of his body.

Some children with cerebral palsy will have problems in dressing and undressing, caused by difficulties in balance, coordination, grasp and maintenance of grasp and in fine manipulation. There may also be difficulties in maintaining attention, perceptual problems, poor body image and difficulties in motor planning. At least some degree of functional independence in dressing skills will be an achievable goal for these children. Parents will need to be able to position their child so that he has a firm, safe base to allow for balance and control of movement. A well-established dressing routine, gradual withdrawal of direct guidance and talking through the dressing sequence, will all help the child to learn the sequences of actions required. The use of clothes which are easier to put on and remove will give him an earlier sense of personal achievement.

The importance of dressing and undressing to the young child with cerebral palsy is the regularity of opportunities that are provided for the child to develop and practise movement and coordination skills and for learning about his body.

Direct teaching of dressing skills may not always be appropriate at this stage as the young child may find this too intrusive, but most parents will need some guidance on how to approach the development of dressing and undressing skills in their child.

3.3.4 BATHING

The infant's independence in the bath is the freedom to sit without parental support, splash and play with bath toys, and enjoy the interaction with his parent as he proceeds with the more serious business of washing. Though young children may dislike certain components of the washing process, bathtime is usually a pleasant, social time for parent and child.

For the child with cerebral palsy, bathtime may not be so much fun. He may be unable to sit unsupported and need to be held by his parent while in the bath. This will be uncomfortable for both, and restrict opportunities for play. Increased tone may make the child difficult to hold and bathtime may become distressing for both parties.

Some children with difficulties in postural control may feel unsafe and insecure in the bath, and their hands used to prop them in sitting will not be available for water play. Negative experiences at bathtime may contribute to a general fear of water and affect the child's future participation in hydrotherapy and swimming.

Parents are likely to need some advice about bathing their child. The use of non-slip mats might be suggested, or the use of a bath seat which will enable the child to play in the water while feeling secure. Bathing can be an excellent opportunity for the child to practise movement, develop body awareness and gain confidence in water.

3.4 Play and learning

Young children spend a substantial proportion of their time engaged in play, and this has a major role in the child's acquisition of knowledge and skills.

Bruner (1972) describes play as providing a forum for the development and practice of behavioural sub-routines that are subsequently integrated into more complex behavioural sequences. Play certainly provides the child with many learning opportunities and access to new experiences, and the essential nature of play with regard to learning can perhaps be seen as the child's involvement in a situation where the process is more important than the product. The function of behaviour is divorced from its normal consequences, and so the stress of anticipated failure or success is reduced (Reynolds, 1976; Sylva *et al.*, 1976). Play can, therefore, be viewed as learning in a less risky situation.

Play is not necessarily separate and distinct from other activities, so, for example, a toddler drinking from his feeder cup may turn it upside down, shake it, watch the liquid escape, and look towards his audience, before resuming drinking. Dressing may involve games of peek-a-boo, and potties may be used as hats. The voluntary nature, spontaneity and intrinsically pleasurable quality of the toddler's play is easily evident to the observer. Play may be initiated by the child or by an adult, but it continues because the child enjoys being a participant.

3.4.1 ATTENTION

The ability to focus, sustain and switch attention is critical to the developing infant's ability to learn through his interactions with his environment. The way in which a child is able to attend in his play changes considerably over his first five years. Cooper *et al.* (1978) describe these changes as a series of stages through which the child's attention becomes more flexible and under his own control. Initially the baby has fleeting attention and is easily distracted. By the second year, attention span has lengthened, allowing for more skilful persistent exploration, but attention tends to be fixed and rigid, as if the infant needs to shut out all external stimuli. At this stage the child can be frustrated and distressed by any interference in his activities. During the third year the child's attention becomes more flexible. He is able to tolerate others' involvement in his play activities, though still very much on his terms. It is not until his fourth year that the child is able to control the focus of his own attention, and up to that point infants are reliant on adults to direct and redirect their attention. For the toddler, cooperative play with an adult sensitive to his intentions in play is possible, but it is not until the fourth and fifth year, when attention control skills are more mature, that cooperative play with peers becomes established.

(a) Implications for the young child with cerebral palsy

(1) The infant's attention control skills may be incompatible with the demands of therapy. Although ostensibly 'play' activities, many therapy

activities designed to improve function are adult-led, and demand cooperation.

External rewards, usually praise or clapping for achievement, may also be used. Many very young children will not have the maturity of attention control to allow them to cope successfully. They may show their frustration by 'tantrums' and some fairly negative behaviour.

Intervention at this stage should reflect the child's developing attention control skills. Activities should be child-initiated and child-led, rewards should be intrinsic and adult involvement should be facilitative rather than intrusive. The adult should assist the child in controlling his attention. Later, as the child matures, he should be able to take on the role of controlling his own attention.

(2) Limited motor skills may necessitate considerable adult involvement in play. This can, however, be facilitative rather than intrusive, and it will be possible, even for a child with severe motor disabilities, to enable him to imitate and lead the play, providing the adult is skilled in interpreting the child's intent.

(3) The infant may, as a consequence of his neurological impairment, have some degree of attention deficit or delay. Most commonly the young child will remain highly distractible and flit from toy to toy in play, or will continue to have single channel, rigid and inflexible attention. Many of these children will also have significant learning difficulties. Play opportunities and therapy activities must reflect the infant's attention level, and should also be designed to facilitate an improvement in length of attention span and in flexibility. Cooper *et al.* (1978) suggest that, for infants in the distractible stage, the learning task should be the major stimulus. Certainly where attention remains rigid and inflexible, giving the child access to highly stimulating toys which give high intrinsic reward seems to be helpful in increasing the child's span of play activity, and self-correcting and intrinsically rewarding activities minimize the distraction and disruption of adult involvement. Adults will need to increase gradually their involvement in the child's play, and build up the child's ability to tolerate adult participation in his activities.

3.4.2   EXPLORATION AND EXPERIMENTATION

The active, inquisitive infant explores his environment and experiments with ways of affecting it. One of the ways in which he learns is by trial and error, adopting initially a fairly random approach, but becoming progressively more systematic in his experiments. Towards the end of the toddler period, he will supplement trial and error approaches with more insightful problem solving. The view that a child learns by acting on and interacting with his environment (Piaget and Inhelder, 1969) has significant implications for those children with cerebral palsy, whose sensori-motor disabilities affect their opportunities to do this. The child who is not independently mobile in the toddler stage, and who cannot use his hands to explore and manipulate objects, is likely to have a passive role in play. He will be stimulated and entertained, moved around by adults, who may also move his limbs to simulate object play experiences, but he is not free to initiate play of his own choosing, or to be active in exploring and experimenting. Children with motor handicaps do present with particular difficulties in understanding spatial relationships (Abercrombie, 1964), which may be consequent on some aspect of their motor experience. Lewis (1987) suggests that differences between children with cerebral palsy indicate that being unable to control movement, as in athetosis or ataxia, has less effect on spatial awareness than if movements are stiff and jerky because of spasticity. Bertenthal and Campos (1987) describe a positive relationship between the infant's active (as opposed to passive) locomotor experience and aspects of his spatial understanding. The relationship between sensori-motor function and cognitive development in children with cerebral palsy can be further complicated by the presence of additional intellectual impairment from damage to associated (non-motor) areas of the brain.

3.4.3 IMITATION

During the preschool period, imitation assumes an increasingly important role in the child's play and learning. Uzgiris (1981) describes the cognitive function of imitation as helping children understand the challenge presented by the model's behaviour, which is just beyond their competence. As the infant matures, there is progressively less dependence on the immediate presence of the model behaviour as the ability to imitate from memory is evidence of emerging symbolic representation. Young children tend to imitate behaviours which have conventional social meaning (Killen and Uzgiris, 1981). They model predominantly on parent behaviours and select from the ongoing stream of behaviours, rather than modelling behaviours deliberately made salient for them. In addition to its role in the acquisition of new practical and social skills, imitation is also regarded as having a role in establishing and sustaining social bonds.

Children with motor difficulties will clearly have problems in imitating motor acts. In addition, however, many children with cerebral palsy have poor body image and spatial skills, which leads to a greater degree of difficulty in copying motor actions than would be predicted from their physical disability alone. These children will not be able to take full advantage of everyday opportunities for learning by copying casually observed actions. Instead, to acquire these skills they will at some stage need a great deal of specific guidance and enhanced feedback, with the activity broken down into very small steps. Young children with cerebral palsy can, however, incorporate imitation into their play and social interaction, provided that the adults are able to interpret these unclear attempts at imitation and respond appropriately.

3.4.4 HELPING THE CHILD WITH CEREBRAL PALSY TO PLAY

(a) Carers' roles

Adult carers will inevitably play an important role in the toy play of a child with a physical disability. In non-disabled infants the major role of the adult carer in play is essentially collaborative and supportive, allowing the child a sense of security during his explorations (Matas *et al.*, 1978). Bruner (1972b) stresses the importance of the carer's role in the young child's play as interpreting the child's intent – identifying the child's intended outcome from play and assisting with those components of a task which a child cannot himself control. He refers to this as 'scaffolding'. Difficulties in mobility and manipulation skills limit the child's initiation and autonomy in play. It is easy for adults to take over and direct his play, removing opportunities for the child to gain enjoyment and knowledge from his own exploring and experimenting. The over-intrusion of adults into play is likely to stress the young child, and where toy play is not enjoyable, the child will focus on aspects of play he enjoys, perhaps social games and rough and tumble, or persist in simpler activities for which his physical abilities are adequate.

Most carers of young children with cerebral palsy will need some help and support from professionals if they are to adopt a facilitative role in their child's play. Good quality parent–infant communication provides the ideal basis for developing play. Interventions designed to enhance early pre-verbal parent–infant interactions should have a positive effect on the parents' ability to interpret their child's intent, and on the child's confidence and persistence in communicating intent and making clear choices. In the early stages of toy play, the parent or carer will need to give the infant time to initiate and respond and give assistance which compensates for the child's physical difficulties, without distracting or taking over the play. As the child matures, adult–infant play can become more cooperative, but can still be essentially child-led. An understanding of learning processes will allow parents to capitalize on learning opportunities in play as they arise and increase the accuracy of their interpretation in their child's play. Moxley-Haegert and Serbin (1983) demonstrated the effectiveness of a developmental education programme for parents which increased the parents' motivation and enhanced the child's skill acquisition.

When the child goes to nursery or playgroup he may still require additional help from an adult, if he is to be actively involved in the play experiences. Here the adult's role will be to enable him to have the same freedom and flexibility in his choice of play as his peers and to allow him to play alongside or cooperatively with other children as appropriate. Once again the adult must adopt a low profile and be facilitative and non-intrusive if the child is to enjoy the experiences of cooperative peer play.

(b)   *Positions for play*

Young children play with toys sitting on the floor or, more rarely, at a table, on their sides or in prone on the floor, kneeling and standing. They change positions frequently and can switch their attention from their play activity to interesting events and interactions around them. Many children with cerebral palsy will need some degree of additional postural support to enable them to have both hands free and functional, and to inhibit involuntary movement and abnormal muscle tone. This will, to some extent, restrict the freedom and flexibility of the child's play, but as far as possible he should have access to a variety of play positions, which enable him to participate in everyday family activities.

It will be the carer's task to position the child for play and, when appropriate, change these positions. For the more mobile child, able to select his own position, this will mean encouraging or persuading him to adopt 'good' positions, probably less comfortable than the positions he prefers, which may not only lead to less than ideal hand function but may also negatively influence the longer term development of good postural control.

Where children need some degree of physical support, carers will need to acquire the techniques for positioning and holding their child in sitting or in standing. To allow for longer play sessions and more independence, they will need to position their child using a variety of special equipment, such as a corner seat, standing frame, or wedge (see Part 3). For children with very little muscle control, the equipment used may be cumbersome and complex, and positioning a child can be difficult and time-consuming.

If parents of children with cerebral palsy are to take on this commitment to facilitate their child's play, they will need to have a clear understanding of the importance of play, not only for learning but also for the child's social development and emotional well-being. Many parents perceive play as peripheral and time-wasting, and those with a child with cerebral palsy will have many competing priorities, such as feeding, and developing their child's mobility and communication. It is also important that the advice given and equipment provided are compatible with the family's lifestyle and routines. Where families spend a lot of time at the homes of grandparents or friends, or the children spend time with a childminder, little use will be made of bulky or heavy equipment left at home. Parents who place a high value on their aesthetically pleasing, coordinated and tidy home are likely to place bulky and ugly equipment in cupboards, from which it may only rarely be retrieved.

The professional's role is, therefore, not only to assess the child's needs for good positions for play, it will also be necessary for them to talk with parents about the role of play and the reasons for 'positioning' the child, and to discover the family's needs and preferences for equipment. Establishing positions where the child can function effectively in play is a relatively straightforward part of the professional's task. Ensuring parental compliance in positioning the child and using equipment is far more complex and challenging. When the child goes to nursery or playgroup he will need access to a similar range of equipment and the adults in these settings must have an understanding of the hows and whys of positioning for play.

(c)   Toys and technology

The young child needs access to age-appropriate toys. It is likely that the child who has difficulties in using his hands in skilful object manipulation will appear to play most easily with toys designed for babies, such as rattles and activity centres, but the perpetuation of play with baby toys into the toddler and preschool period both reinforces the image of the infant with cerebral palsy as a baby, and will deprive the child of access to playthings which reflect and extend his growing knowledge of his social and physical world.

As play becomes increasingly sophisticated, the infant requires toys which allow him to explore the functional relationships between objects, such as size, shape and colour. Initially he also needs toys which represent his world in a realistic way, e.g. dolls, cars, cups, telephones, as it is not until later that he will be able to improvise in pretend play, by using objects which bear little or no resemblance to the real thing.

The facilitative role of parents will be important in enabling children to play with age-appropriate toys. This is particularly appropriate for pretend play, but it is also essential for the young child to have some play which is independent of adults, and which gives him an experience of mastery. Intrinsic reward is an essential component of young childrens' play (Donaldson, 1978). The child with cerebral palsy, however, is likely to need to make a much greater effort than his peers to achieve the same reward.

The task of parents in collaboration with professionals is to find toys which are appropriate to the child's cognitive ability, are easy for the child to manipulate, and give a high intrinsic reward. Many commercially available toys which parents can obtain from a toy library will be suitable. Fat crayons which mark easily on paper will make drawing more rewarding; bricks which stick together easily will encourage early constructional play; and postboxes which give an auditory reward will encourage a greater degree of persistence. It may also be possible to adapt toys to make them easier to hold and manipulate, and the use of non-slip mats or tables with cups will ensure that toys stay within reach of the immobile child.

A few children with cerebral palsy will have such limited control of movement that either they will be unable to participate actively in object play, or the movements they are able to make may limit their play to very basic holding, shaking, banging actions. The task for these children will be to enable them to use any purposeful movement that they have to affect their environment in a way which is consistent with their cognitive development, rather than their motor competence. Both switch operated action toys and the computer will provide the child with a high reward for his action, and will be instrumental in his gaining an understanding of cause and effect, and in developing switch access skills. This will be essential to the child with very severe motor disability, who will later need to use more sophisticated educational technology, operate an electric wheelchair or access alternative communication and environmental control systems. Once children understand the link between their action and toy/computer operation, they can be further challenged by the use of more than one switch for different toys or functions, or the directional use of a joystick.

(d) Gross motor play

In running, jumping, climbing and pushing himself around on trundle toys, the young child is practising and perfecting his gross motor skills, learning about the spatial relationships of his world, and acquiring a few bruises. Rough and tumble, usually with adults at this age, is also a component of the child's play repertoire.

Children who have no independent mobility, or whose mobility is severely restricted, will not have access to these play experiences unless it is possible to provide them with early access to an electrically operated wheelchair, or to a trolley or other mobility aid which he can propel physically. Even those children who have some mobility will appreciate the use of a trundle toy, which will increase their enjoyment of movement and exploration of their surroundings.

The major issues for discussion between therapists and parent will be the extent to which the use of a mobility aid or trundle toy will facilitate or impede the development of good postural control and movement patterns, and whether a mobility aid or trundle toy will encourage or discourage the child in his attempts to be independently mobile. There is no evidence to support the idea that early use of mobility aids in play reduces motivation for independent mobility. An aid or toy supplied for play need not be used throughout the child's day, but can be limited to play sessions. It can be argued that enjoyable experiences of mobility in play will increase rather than decrease the child's general motivation to be independently mobile.

Allowing a child with poor balance and inadequate saving reactions to climb and move around on his trundle toy involves a degree of risk. Letting him do this in the company of boisterous mobile toddlers is unthinkable to many parents. There is also a tendency to handle the child with cerebral palsy like a china doll, and he misses the social and physical experiences of being thrown around in rough and tumble.

The close involvement of parents in their child's physical therapy should help them overcome their fears about handling him in this sort of play. They may need some advice on positioning and holding him, so that he can enjoy movement in rough and tumble, and they may also need to discuss the risks involved in their child's participation in gross motor play, particularly with peers. The difference between protection and overprotection is one of individual judgement, and parents will need to be able to balance risks against the social and cognitive benefits of early autonomy in locomotion.

3.5 Movement

3.5.1 POSTURAL CONTROL AND MOBILITY

The basis of voluntary movement is normal muscle tone, which allows normal postural control, integrated primary responses and the slowly emerging development of equilibrium and righting reactions. The combination of these factors allows the child better coordinated movements with more discreet motor patterns carried out with precision, the child is therefore not only able to walk and run but to stop and start quickly and negotiate obstacles. As the child develops, he is able to increase his repertoire of more highly skilled movement, and so build up the number of his available postural sets. His increasingly reliable balance reactions give him a secure base from which to move and allow him to function better against gravity without falling. This leads to a greater security and enjoyment of movement with more mature sensory motor experiences.

The child's early impulses, such as casting objects and constantly moving backwards and forwards to reinforce the sensation of movement, are slowly inhibited to socially acceptable levels as the child is able to be more selective as to which stimuli he responds to. He has also to be able to do more than one thing at a time, for example, carry an object while walking. The child begins to be able to plan a sequence of physical activities, which will enable him to achieve a more complex aim, for example, rising from the floor to sitting on a chair. The child at this stage enjoys physical activities and his first interaction with his peers is often through a physical medium. The child becomes able to reinforce his personality physically, for example, by moving away from challenge, thereby aiding his emotional and social development.

Children learn about the environment by physically manoeuvring themselves upstairs, down slopes, pushing heavy objects and feeling the effects of gravity and external forces upon them. By moving and coordinating the body, the child develops a body image and concept of the body shape and size. Physical endurance and strength gradually increase with time, many new skills are learnt on a trial and error basis, and the child becomes able to modify and adapt his existing sensori-motor experiences with the knowledge and memory of past experiences. The more the movements are repeated, the less effort is required, as the movement becomes more automatic and less volitional.

(a) *The impact of cerebral palsy*

The child with cerebral palsy experiences great difficulty in coordinating and executing movements, owing primarily to an alteration in his normal postural control mechanism (Bobath and Bobath, 1975), the persistence of pathological and retained primary responses, and the diminished or absent equilibrium and righting reactions.

The lesion in the brain usually manifests itself by an alteration in muscle tone, either hypertonia, with spasticity, or hypotonia, or indeed fluctuating tone as in children with ataxia or athetosis. The distribution of this abnormal tone depends primarily on the site of the initial lesion in the brain, and the condition can be further classified according to the area of the body affected (see below). Tone is also a very variable phenomenon and is influenced by many factors such as effort, fear, pain, position, all of which may aggravate the increase in tone and distribution of it, whereas appropriate postures and patterns of movement, techniques of handling and weight-bearing, may 'normalize' the muscle tone. The persistence of pathological reflexes, such as asymmetric tonic neck reflex, Galant, etc., may lead to stereotyped motor responses arresting the child's development and, if left un-treated, leading on to fixed deformities. The equilibrium and righting reactions needed for moving against gravity may be slow to emerge or absent, making balance and the realignment of the body and reinstate-ment of the stable posture difficult. The alteration in muscle tone often manifests itself in abnormal co-contraction – this is the fine balance between agonist/antagonist, which allows a smooth graded movement to occur; it also allows proximal stability so that distally finer move-ments can be carried out. The co-contraction is either excessive if the tone is generally increased (spastic), fluctuating (athetoid), or diminished (ataxic). Stability is either very hard to achieve, as in chil-dren with athetosis and ataxia, or excessive, as in spasticity, allowing very little mobility.

The child often lacks inhibition of movement and reacts to a stimulus every time with the result that his movements are very predictable and stereotyped. His sensori-motor experiences are therefore very limited and abnormal. When the child tries to move he will try to use these patterns as these are all he knows, thereby reinforcing them. The child has very few and abnormal postural sets. Gross motor planning is therefore very hard to achieve, and movements can only be done in a few abnormal ways. Poor equilibrium and righting reactions mean the child is very unstable against gravity, and often falls without the ability either to stop himself or protect himself once fallen. The child may have no stable base from which to move and lack the ability to regain his stability once his equilibrium is disturbed. Movement is therefore not always a pleasurable experience, and involves a great deal of effort. Frustration compounds the problem, and all these factors only serve further to increase tone and to make further movement even more difficult; efforts to do so become counter-productive. Therefore the child is left with very poor sensory experience and may rely heavily on his parents to provide these for him. This physical dependence will make separation from parents even more difficult later.

One consequence of the above is that parents may tend to over-protect their child, and inadvertently prevent the child from gaining necessary experience to learn about equilibrium and righting reactions. As the child is often so physically dependent on his parents, his emotional and social development will be slow to emerge, and his early interaction with his peers delayed. The body concept, spatial relation-ships and visuo-motor development will be affected in a similar way.

The child at this stage needs to be encouraged to be as physically active and get as much enjoyment out of movement as possible. The aim of physical intervention is to facilitate more normal movement patterns, and to try to inhibit the use of primitive stereotyped reflexes. This is an interactive process between the child and whoever is handling him at the time. Control over the movement is gradually handed over to the child. The child's role, therefore, is not passive, and he should take as much responsibility over his physical skills as possible. This need should be frequently re-assessed and support withdrawn as felt appropriate. The child will always revert back to his well-established stereotyped movement patterns when angry and frustrated, which can be seen, for example, in total extension of the body initiated by hand and shoulder retraction, which a normal child also shows. The child with cerebral palsy, however, should be dissuaded from perseverating in these movements, as they will further hamper his progress. The child continuing to extend in such a fashion will not be able to sit or stand independently. Such long-term aims, of course, will not be understood by the child, and so play and movement should be so structured as to enable the child to succeed in the task with the minimum of frustration.

The child needs to take responsibility for his own body and not rely entirely on others to do things for him. Simple tasks like dressing should involve the child in lifting up his foot to put on a sock, while sitting on his parent's lap with minimal support while his shoes are put on. These activities will help him control his own body movements, while he is also reinforcing his balance reaction.

The child's primary disability may be compounded by the interplay between the disability and environmental influences, thus giving rise to secondary handicaps. For example, normal social skills may be impeded by slow motor development. The young child who is unable to move quickly cannot participate in games of chase, or resolve a conflict over a snatched toy by pursuing the culprit. Mobility opens up choice for the non-handicapped child. It is the key to increased independence. Children in nursery defy their teachers by moving away. Mobility aids such as sticks, rollators or other adapted equipment enable the child with cerebral palsy to retain a certain independence and facilitate motor development.

The question of powered mobility may be raised at the preschool stage. A study examining the correlates of powered mobility and self-initiated exploration in six children with locomotor difficulties indicated that the provision of powered wheelchairs facilitated longer periods spent in object play. However, firm conclusions cannot be drawn from this study, which was designed only as a preliminary investigation.

Further research is required into the accessibility of buildings for wheelchairs, the importance of parental views and whether the motivation to walk is extinguished or decreased if the child is using a wheelchair or other mobility aid at an early age.

3.5.2 FINE MOTOR SKILLS

The young child's development of fine motor skills is influenced by his gross motor development. When he begins to walk and hold his arms in the high guard position, and concentrates totally on maintaining his balance, fine motor skills appear to regress. It is, however, not long before he has sufficient stability and confidence in gross motor skills to allow him to manipulate and hold objects again.

The toddler is able to combine walking with holding objects, and is able to use his hands in exploration and manipulation while standing. This opens up a wide range of new opportunities for developing and practising fine motor skills. The toddler's movements become increasingly controlled and precise. He becomes a skilled tool user and learns to coordinate the use of both hands together. Fine motor ability is essential to the child's developing independence and is important in his play and learning.

(a) The impact of cerebral palsy

Many children with cerebral palsy are likely to have difficulty in developing fine motor skills, because of the involvement of one or both upper limbs. They may have problems in strength, precision, range and control of movement and also receive attenuated or distorted sensory feedback. In addition to these primary factors, children with cerebral palsy may also experience secondary limitations in opportunities to develop and practise hand skills, because of the involvement of their arms in maintaining balance in sitting and standing and of their extensive use of their arms in assisting mobility in crawling or in holding on to furniture or a rollator. Also, children with diplegia and spina bifida may show depressed manipulative ability in using their hands when these have been involved for primary mobility or for support with walking aids, rather than in conventional manual exploration.

Good distal control relies on good proximal control. All children who have difficulties in maintaining good balance and posture in sitting and standing will have even greater difficulties in hand control.

A small number of children with cerebral palsy experience a persistence of reflexes, such as the asymmetric tonic neck. This may lead to a more general asymmetry, and to poor development of the midline concept. This in turn will adversely affect the development of eye–hand coordination and bimanual dexterity.

The greater effort required to manipulate objects with just one hand may give rise to associated reactions in the other, and it may become increasingly more difficult to involve this hand in bimanual tasks. Fine motor skills will be delayed, and some children will adopt alternative strategies, often using their mouth instead of a hand. Fine motor skills require good proprioceptive ability in the upper limbs. One of the ways in which children develop this is through weight-bearing; first in pushing up in prone, then in propping up sitting and in crawling. Where infants with cerebral palsy have not been able to experience weight-bearing through their arms, they are likely to have a diminished awareness of the position of their arms in space.

Limited or inappropriate experiences in weight-bearing may also contribute to hypersensitivity in the hands, so that the child will find touching, holding, manipulating and exploring with his hands unpleasant, and will avoid tactile experiences, or limit himself to a few familiar objects, with a consequent detrimental effect on the acquisition of fine motor dexterity.

(b)   Intervention

During the early years, when much of the emphasis in therapy is likely to be on the development of mobility, it will be necessary to focus specifically on facilitating the development of fine motor skills, even in those children whose cerebral palsy does not primarily affect their upper limbs. The first task will be to find positions in sitting and in standing which will give the child good proximal stability, and allow his hands to be free for object manipulation (see Part 3).

Rather than restrict 'hand skill practice' to a specific table and chair and a set of toys, a variety of easily accessible positions will allow the infant with cerebral palsy access to the many everyday situations in which his non-handicapped contemporaries enjoy developing and practising their fine motor skills.

Initially, children with cerebral palsy should be encouraged to play in midline. This will maximize eye–hand coordination and inhibit asymmetric tonic neck reflexes. Eventually, objects can be placed to the side so that the child has to cross the midline.

Where hypersensitivity is a problem, it will be necessary to provide carefully graded tactile experiences so that gradual desensitization can take place. The child can also be facilitated from the shoulders rather than having objects placed in his hands.

4 The school age child

4.1 The transition to school

4.1.1 FAMILY ISSUES

A child's starting school is an event of major significance in the life of the family. For most parents it is essentially positive, associated with expectations of the child's future and an appraisal of their own achievement so far as parents. Where a child has a disability, starting school may have a different significance. Farber (1975) suggests that families appear not to make one simple major adaptation following diagnosis/disclosure of their child's disability, but rather to make a series of minimal adaptations, changing only so far as circumstances compel them at the time. The child's starting school involves the parents in a reassessment of the impact of the child's disability on both her own and the family's future. Even families who have had good information and counselling and have coped well and worked positively in their child's therapy may not have fully acknowledged the permanence and seriousness of their child's disability. The emotional distress which some families experience during this period sometimes surprises both the parents themselves and the professionals. A child's transfer from primary to secondary school may similarly be a time of painful reassessment for parents. Most parents will need some degree of support during and after their child's entry into school. Some parents will have particular needs for counselling during these transitional periods.

The sense of loss and the vacuum experienced, at least fleetingly, by most parents when their child starts school can be much more significant when the child has cerebral palsy. The parent has spent much more time and energy than average in physical care, has become skilled in managing the child and is a 'key worker' in the child's therapy and teaching programmes. Parents may find it particularly difficult to hand over responsibility for day-to-day care of their child to school staff. In taking on the traditional role of parents with regard to the school, they may feel excluded from their child's management and therapy.

Parents will also lose the regular contacts with therapists and teachers who have been working with them in the preschool period. Some of these professionals will have been regular home visitors and will have taken on the role of supportive friends. There is, however, much that can be done by both preschool services and schools to make the transition easier. The preschool professionals can continue to have contact with the parent during the child's first term at school, perhaps facilitating contact and communication between home and school. Schools can involve parents from an early stage, seeking their advice on aspects of the child's feeding etc. Parents may be enabled to stay with their child for some part of the school day and encouraged to participate in classroom activities during the school week. Where the child is at a special school, there should be sufficient flexibility to meet parents' individual needs. In mainstream schools it will not be desirable to make the child look different by having her parent in the classroom, but teachers can make use of arrival and departure times for talking to parents.

4.1.2   THE CHILD IN SCHOOL

School is the location in which much of a child's learning and development will take place. Selection of school and preparation for school is particularly important for the child with cerebral palsy, whose academic and social progress may, at some stage in her educational career, be complicated if not severely compromised by her disabilities.

(a)   Mainstream or special school?

The education of children with physical handicaps has traditionally taken place in special schools, where the concentration of resources and trained staff allows for levels of attention which are not normally available in mainstream schools. This centralization of resources and the development of expertise and excellence are the most compelling arguments in favour of separate special schools. Many children with cerebral palsy will have special educational needs related to their movement difficulties or their learning or emotional problems, but a need for special educational provision is not synonymous with a need for a segregated special school. The growth of commitment within the health and social services to the integration of the individual with a disability into her community has been paralleled by a change in ideology, policy and finally practice in education. Integration is the new orthodoxy, such that special schools must now justify their existence (Hodgson *et al.*, 1984). The prevailing assumption enshrined in legislation is that pupils should be considered first for placement in a mainstream school, and only when this is problematic should special school placement be made.

For parents of an individual child, the choice of educational provision will be constrained not just by the child's disability, but more crucially by the policy, practice and resources of the local education authority. In a study of integrated provision for children with special needs throughout Britain, Hegarty *et al.* (1981) concluded that integration is possible to a far greater extent than is currently the practice. Practice in integration is diverse: in some authorities children with significant physical disabilities will be educated within special schools, whereas in others, children with similar needs will be offered some degree of integrated provision. Hegarty (1982) concludes: 'as long as some pupils attend special schools when their peers elsewhere, with comparable special needs, receive satisfactory education in ordinary schools, there are grounds for disquiet.'

Provision for children with physical disabilities and with mild to moderate learning difficulties is often made in units attached to mainstream schools. Units provide a separate base for the children with special needs. Participation of most children in the school can vary between almost complete separation, where children meet only for assemblies (even having separate playgrounds for protection), to extensive participation in mainstream classroom and social activities.

Jones (1983) describes such units as a 'Limpet Model': 'like limpets on a ship, children in a unit attached to a mainstream school will have "waves of normality wash over them". Secure and cossetted in their special education lifebelts, they float around ordinary schools like observers to the mainstream scene.'

Certainly social integration is more difficult for children in a unit. They are not from the neighbourhood and are identifiable as members of a large group of children with disabilities. Hegarty *et al.*'s (1981) findings regarding children with physical disabilities in a unit confirmed that peer friendships between disabled and able-bodied children were the exception rather than the norm. Nevertheless, children who had transferred from special school to a mainstream unit were essentially positive in their evaluation. They valued the increased independence and enhanced social and academic opportunities.

Decisions about meeting a child's special educational needs are not restricted to the preschool period. Some children who cope well in mainstream school may experience difficulties as the social and academic or perhaps physical demands of school increase. Conversely, initial decisions to place a child in special provision may be reconsidered, either in view of the child's progress or because of changes in education policy. Regular review of the child's individual needs remains essential, whether she is in a mainstream or special school.

(b) Which mainstream school?

Where a child has a disability, the parents' role in choosing a mainstream school is vital. Most parents will opt for a local school enabling the child to establish and maintain friendships with a neighbourhood peer group. If the neighbourhood school is not ideal because of other considerations, location should still be a factor in selecting an alternative. Will the child be able to get to school independently when she is mature enough? Can she walk there? Are there steep hills or main roads to cross? Is there a bus link?

Some thought should also be given to ease of access of school friends who live in the school neighbourhood. A school's buildings may also be important. A child with a mild physical disability who is slow in mobility or unsteady on her feet is likely to be disadvantaged and vulnerable in a building with long distances between classrooms, steep stairs, or sloping playgrounds. Consideration should also be given to the suitability of buildings to which the child will progress, so that unnecessary disruption of the child's peer friendships will be minimized.

If necessary, transport could be provided, buildings could be adapted and ancillary help could be made available. School ethos and staff attitudes, while not immutable, may not be so readily amenable to change. Hegarty (1982) describes the enthusiasm of the head, and the head's ability to enlist the cooperation of staff, as crucial factors in successful integration, and clearly a school ethos which values children irrespective of their abilities and attainments will be linked to successful integration of a child with special needs. Where a school has accommodated a child with special needs in the past, it should be possible to discover in what ways the curriculum had been adapted, and how support was given within the classroom. This will give an indication of the school's flexibility. Evidence of the school's ability to involve and work with other professionals and involvement of parents will indicate the school's openness and ability to communicate effectively.

(c) Supporting the child in mainstream school

The support strategies adopted for a particular child will depend not only on her individual needs as determined by the nature and severity of her disability, and their potential influence on her physical, social and academic integration, but also on the characteristics and needs of the school, including factors already outlined in the previous section.

(i) Staff preparation and training   This should take place prior to the child's entry to school to ensure a high degree of initial success. Staff who have contact with the child will need to have a clear understanding of the nature of her disability and how it may affect her in school. They would need to know, for example, that, although the child can walk competently, she tires easily and will find long walks on school outings difficult. An awareness that a child's difficulties in writing, drawing and numbers are related to perceptual difficulties rather than simply motor problems, or more general intellectual impairment, will enable the staff to respond more sensitively and minimize the child's experience of failure and stress. Where positioning or seating are important, a knowledge of 'why' is more likely to lead to staff compliance with advice. Staff will need to be confident in handling and operating apparatus and equipment. When a child has a communication difficulty, staff must be enabled to interpret her communication. This will range from listening and 'tuning in' to her speech, to using a sophisticated alternative communication system. Staff must also be able to facilitate the child's communication with peers.

There are many staff in a school who will need additional knowledge and skills in order to respond effectively to a child's special needs. People who supervise during lunchtime and playtime, for example, will need an understanding of eating and mobility difficulties. Most staff preparation can occur informally, with meetings between school staff, parents and other specialist professionals, although some members of staff will benefit from attending courses.

(ii) Building adaptations, aids, etc.   Building adaptations such as ramps, rails, toilet adaptations and lifts, will require some financial commitment from the education authority or other equivalent funding body. In some cases this may be considerable, and in most instances the child will need to transfer between first, middle and secondary schools, these costs will be replicated. With the exception of lifts, however, most adaptations require minimal maintenance and will make the school more accessible to others with physical disabilities.

The purpose of building adaptations is usually to allow access. This will include access to classrooms, toilets, dining room and playground, and also to certain areas of the school for specific curriculum activities (art room, science laboratories, cookery room). Older children will usually be required to move around the school for many different subjects. Where costs of providing unrestricted access within school are prohibitive and/or where finance is restricted, alternatives may have to be considered. It may be possible to alter timetables and relocate activities, or a non-teaching assistant could be introduced specifically to facilitate access where this is difficult.

Aids such as wheelchairs, walking frames, word processors and communication boards will have to be physically accommodated within the school. Where can a wheelchair be stored when not in use? How can a word processor be accessible but safe from other inquisitive children?

(iii) Specialist support   The primary function of the professional support services – health, social service and education – is to support the child's development and quality of experience through the agency of the primary carers. In the preschool period this is usually the parents' task. At school age the teacher also must be considered as having this role. Many teachers will have had neither personal experience of working with people with disabilities nor any specific training regarding education of children with special needs. Thus, although there may be a willingness to learn and adapt, the support agencies may well have to approach the problem from a fairly basic level, not assuming any degree of sophistication. In sharing knowledge and expertise and in advising the teachers who are to implement 'programmes' or 'strategies' it must be recognized that teachers may not have the skill base that the parent has acquired, nor a knowledge of the specialist language or jargon.

As most professionals have time constraints because of caseloads, it is useful to maximize their effective support by identifying 'key workers' within the child's school. At primary school this will usually be the child's teacher (who will change each year, involving retraining) and possibly an ancillary worker. At secondary level this may well be the 'special needs coordinator' or support teacher. In some primary schools this role may be assumed by the headteacher.

This designated individual can facilitate the integration of outside support and expertise into school by liaison between school staff, parents and outside professionals, convening and organizing multi-disciplinary meetings, reviews and reassessments, ensuring that information is appropriately disseminated and that training needs are identified and met.

Careful planning and negotiation should avoid conflicts between school staff and professionals with no mainstream education background. The latter may have little appreciation of a teacher's tasks in a large classroom and may interpret limited knowledge, time and resources as lack of interest or non-compliance. Similarly, teachers may perceive the professionals as having unrealistic expectations.

(iv) Additional staffing Where the child has needs for practical assistance, guidance, support or supervision, which cannot be met by the school's existing staff, provision of an extra teacher or, more commonly, a non-teaching assistant may meet these needs.

There are many roles which can be taken on by a non-teaching assistant to enable a child with a disability to function as independently as possible and participate fully within the curriculum and social life of the school. Help can be provided with mobility and everyday activities such as eating, dressing and toileting. Additional supervision can allow a child to participate in activities that would otherwise be considered too risky, e.g. cookery, PE, the playground. The non-teaching assistant may attend the child's therapy sessions, continue practice of therapy programmes, or be responsible for the child's integration into school activities. She may also take some responsibility for the care and use of the child's aids and equipment in school. Within the classroom help may be given with activities which are difficult, e.g. taking notes.

Where a child has additional problems or learning difficulties, additional individual help may enable her to continue to learn within a mainstream class. A non-teaching assistant or additional teacher can also be used to allow the class teacher to spend more time with the child with special needs.

Children's needs for extra individual help will change as they progress through school. Most children will become increasingly independent and begin to take on for themselves the tasks of the non-teaching assistant, e.g. dressing after PE and toiletting. In some instances, needs for additional help will increase as buildings or the curriculum become more demanding. It is essential that the right amount of individual help is available from the start, that it is used appropriately, and that its use is reviewed and monitored. Too little help will cause a child to struggle and fail, too much and the child's independence will be restricted, her sense of achievement and self-mastery diminished, and she will be unnecessarily presented to her peers as different and dependent.

(v) Parental involvement Good communication with parents and parental involvement in the life of the school is regarded as sound educational practice. Schools vary in their relationships with parents, some are minimal and formalized in open days and through parent governers, while other schools, particularly primary schools, welcome parents into the classroom and encourage joint working between home and school.

The expertise of a parent of a child with special needs may be considerable, and should be valued and respected. Parents should be involved as part of the team of school staff and other specialist professionals, and continue to feel involved in the planning of the child's therapy. Regular communication is essential, but participation in classroom activities should be organized so that the child is not made to appear even more different by being the only one to have a parent in class. Where the child is not skilled in communication, a home–school book may ensure a link between parents and teachers, and provide the context in which the parent can interpret the child's communication.

Hegarty (1982) suggests that parents benefit from seeing their child's special needs met in an ordinary school where the child engages in activities alongside non-disabled peers: 'When this happens they are less likely to perceive their child in terms of the handicapped identity ascribed by society, and may be helped to see him or her as a precious individual who happens to have special needs.'

(vi) Curriculum A mainstream school curriculum may require some modification to meet the needs of a child with cerebral palsy. Some children will have limited curriculum access skills, e.g. spoken or written communication, or may need extra time, or have to make much greater effort to achieve the same goals as their peers. The child may also be withdrawn for therapy. These children should be able to follow a basically normal timetable, but some modifications will be necessary to allow for omissions or supplementary activities.

Where the child has significant learning difficulties, these modifications may need to be much more substantial. Extra time may need to be spent in acquiring basic curriculum access skills (literacy and numeracy), but it should still be possible for the child to follow the normal curriculum. Careful scrutiny of the curriculum will be essential in planning for the integration of a child into a school.

4.2 Interaction

4.2.1 SOCIAL AND EMOTIONAL DEVELOPMENT

(a) Peer relationships

During the school years, relationships with peers become increasingly important. Peer friendships are regarded as making a major contribution to the development of social competency and mature social behaviours in children (Hartup, 1978). Peer relationships are also considered crucial in the learning of role taking, different perspectives, empathy and in enabling children to establish appropriate and socially acceptable boundaries for aggressive feelings and behaviours (Gottman *et al.*, 1975; Hartup, 1974). Poor peer relationships in childhood are associated with later mental health difficulties (Rutter, 1985).

Some children with cerebral palsy will have significant difficulties in making friends and establishing a positive role within their peer group. Many of these children will already be disadvantaged before starting school. Difficulties in early relationships with carers and restricted preschool peer socialization will not provide an optimal foundation for school age socialization. Movement and communication difficulties may have restricted social interaction and participation and may continue to do so at school.

As well as secondary factors, some individuals may have intrinsic learning difficulties and may be delayed in acquiring the social knowledge and skills essential to successful peer interactions. The child may also have particular difficulties in social and emotional relationships. Children whose physical disability is associated with 'brain damage' are more likely to have emotional difficulties and later psychiatric problems than other children with equivalent physical disabilities (Rutter *et al.*, 1970).

By school age, the child will face further hurdles. Her peers will take on the values of their parents and are likely to adopt a negative view of differences in her appearance and behaviour. Peer group rejection is likely, particularly in response to perceived social and intellectual deficits, rather than to a physical disability, but the child with cerebral palsy may well experience social isolation and rejection in her school years. In addition, friendships are based on shared interests, mutual esteem and reciprocity. Friends tend to be, in many respects, similar (Hartup, 1983). Even without peer group rejection, the child with cerebral palsy may not have friends (Anastasiow, 1984), and may have a low status within her peer group.

Children's self-concept becomes more sophisticated during the early school years and they are increasingly influenced by others' perceptions of them. They will also become more aware of the implications of their disability or underachievements. The child with cerebral palsy is likely to have been aware of her disability and her difference from others prior to starting school, but it seems that it is not until the early school years that negative effects on self-esteem become evident (Teplin *et al.*, 1981).

(b)   Intervention

One response to the possibility of peer group rejection, and social isolation and its negative effects on self-esteem, has been to protect the child by maintaining her within a segregated special school. Although for some children special school may be necessary for practical, educational or financial reasons, there is no evidence that it will protect the child from the negative consequences of poor peer relationships. There are indications that, for children with cerebral palsy, relationships with non-handicapped peers are positive factors in emerging self-concept and that the maintenance of relationships with non-handicapped peers is a crucial factor in the later coping ability of these children (Minde *et al.*, 1972; Minde, 1978).

Where integration is not possible in school, efforts can be made to maintain and develop a child's relationships with non-handicapped peers at home, in the neighbourhood and by participation in integrated clubs and youth organizations. The physical presence and participation of a child with cerebral palsy in a group of non-disabled peers will not, in itself, guarantee positive peer relationships, but can be regarded as an essential prerequisite for the acquisition of peer-related social skills.

The more challenging environment of an integrated setting offers opportunities for observational learning and increases the likelihood of receiving adaptive consequences from interactions with peers (Guralnick, 1981). Children's social behaviours can be facilitated by the modelling of social behaviours by their more sociable peers (Field *et al.*, 1981) and children whose skills are mildly delayed show improvements in developmental functioning and appropriate social behaviours consequent on their interactions with more competent children (Guralnick, 1981). In addition, interactions are least likely to be successful when both members of a dyad have communication difficulties (Beveridge and Brinker, 1980). Thus an integrated setting will allow not only for social learning but also for increased feedback from social interactions. It is also possible for adults to encourage, prompt and reward appropriate social behaviours (Timm *et al.*, 1979) or to manage the learning environment so as to establish cooperative play and learning experiences (Slavin, 1980).

Some individual children may beneift from specific tutoring in social skills. This may include increasing their ability to read social cues, to develop positive social behaviours and appropriate responses to social approaches (Hops and Greenwood, 1981).

Some thought about the child's image and appearance may also facilitate integration into the peer group. Dress and possessions should be age-appropriate and suggest competence. Where a child has difficulty manipulating buttons and zips, elasticated waistbands on trousers or skirts seem practicable, but discrete use of Velcro fastenings should enable the child to wear clothing similar to that of the peer group. Where a child drools excessively when concentrating, time and effort spent teaching a child to monitor this and wipe appropriately will avoid the ignominy of bibs or wet shirts.

Aids and equipment can similarly be positive and 'high tech' rather than shabby and medical. They can be used to engage peer interest and active involvement.

Finally children will be influenced by the attitudes and behaviours of adults towards the child with a disability. Teachers (and adults in a similar role) can also undertake some tutoring of the peer group – enabling them to understand the child's difficulties, access her communication system and help with mobility. They can also counsel children when there are problems or potential difficulties. Positive attitudes and sensitivity on the part of the adults can do much to facilitate the social integration of the child with a disability and prevent the damaging consequences of rejection and isolation.

4.2.2   COMMUNICATION IN THE SCHOOL AGE CHILD

The school age child is expected to be able to communicate fully and to use language to interact with family and peers, teachers and others. Language, spoken or written, is the main medium through which school work is conducted. It becomes increasingly important as the child grows older and educational assessments tend to be based on verbal tasks.

As well as verbal development, the school age child should have grasped many of the rules of social interaction, for example, acceptable strategies for initiating, maintaining and terminating conversations. Language and communication skills are also used in the child's social life outside school, in formal play sessions with other children, and organized activities such as Woodcraft, Cubs, Brownies, etc.

The type of experiences a child with cerebral palsy may have in school depends on the severity with which her disorder affects her oral musculature and on the type of school she attends. There are three broad possibilities:

1. Mild difficulties in mainstream education.
2. Moderate to severe difficulties in mainstream, plus or minus an alternative communication system.
3. Moderate to severe difficulties in a non-integrated setting plus or minus an alternative communication system.

(1) Children with mildly affected oral musculature who attend a mainstream school may require some help with communication, language and speech skills. A degree of dysarthria may result in inaccurate production of speech sounds, especially in rapid speech

or long sentences, resulting in varying degrees of intelligibility. This may affect their being understood by teachers and peers on occasion, but the more serious implication is that the accurate timing required for social interaction may be affected. It is important for schoolchildren to feel themselves accepted by their peers, and communication affected in this way may add extra stress to the child in school.

Speech therapy may help the child ameliorate some of the oral difficulties, and maximize potential for intelligibility, but it is also important for all the staff and parents involved with the child to realize this potential problem and foster relationships between the child with cerebral palsy and other children. Relationships fostered in this way will then be easier to encourage outside school.

(2) Children attending a mainstream school who have more severe difficulties may need to use a sign or symbol system to augment their communication. Criteria for the choice of a communication system and the implications of its use are discussed more fully in Chapter 13, but it is important to note here that children will need help in using their system at school and cannot be expected to integrate its use with their school friends and teachers spontaneously. As with children not requiring the use of an alternative system, parents and teachers should be ready to foster relationships actively between children with cerebral palsy and their classmates.

It will be difficult for a child using an alternative system to initiate conversations unless she has some acceptable way of attracting the attention of the people she wishes to communicate with. This should be given urgent consideration by those involved with the child, who may otherwise find efficient but not particularly socially acceptable ways of attracting attention, e.g. groaning.

(3) The child using an alternative system in a non-integrated setting may also experience difficulties in initiating and maintaining inter-action with other children and with teachers. The other children may not be using the same system, may not be able to achieve physical proximity for conversation easily, and given the difficulties involved and the effort required to communicate, many children may lose the motivation to communicate with each other, preferring to interact with adults who can put a more sophisticated interpretation upon their efforts. It is very important, therefore, that teachers and parents are aware of this, and attempt to facilitate relationships and interaction in school and at home. It may be necessary for someone to act an interpreter's role for some time at the beginning of relationships, gradually withdrawing help as the children become more competent in communicating with each other.

Communication aids, whether sophisticated micro-electronic equipment or symbol or letter boards, must always be available for the child every hour of the day. Although the speech therapist will assist in the child's development of the use of these items, it is important that their use is not restricted to speech therapy sessions, or to certain times during the day at the discretion of the adults involved.

4.3   Independence

By school age, children generally have acquired the practical skills underlying dressing, washing, eating and toiletting. Initially they may need some prompting and supervision, but very soon are expected to take on the responsibility for these self-care activities within school. A child with cerebral palsy is likely to lack the basic skills, or be slower or less precise in their execution. The child's needs for continued learning of personal independence skills will not be shared by her peers. In special schools 'daily living skills' can be a part of the curriculum taught in timetabled sessions and practised during daily routines. Teachers and occupational therapists can work collaboratively on these activities. In mainstream schools, withdrawal may be an option either for individual tuition or where the school has a unit for group sessions. This will, however, restrict the child's participation in other aspects of the curriculum. As regards day-to-day practice of these activities in a mainstream setting, priority is likely to be given to function and speed. The child must be enabled to dress and undress quickly for PE sessions, swimming etc. The child must be clean and neat (or at least as clean and neat as her peers), able to eat and drink adequately without mess, and be continent without accidents. A careful assessment of what help will be needed if the child is to function effectively in school will be essential. The occupational therapist can give advice to school staff on the use of aids and adaptations, and on techniques and strategies which will enable them to help the child efficiently, and allow the child to continue to learn and develop independence. Personal independence skills are, of course, an integral part of home as well as school life. Any teaching of daily living skills should involve parents as well as school staff. For children at mainstream school the home, during school holidays when there is no time pressure, may be the optimal setting in which to learn and practise new skills. There should be a regular review of children's needs for assistance, and for training in personal independence skills as they mature.

Within school, dressing may be facilitated by the use of loose fitting clothing and the adaptation of difficult fastenings with Velcro. The child's clothing should be age-appropriate and indistinguishable from that of peers.

For toiletting, the major concerns will be mobility, access and handling clothing. An age-appropriate degree of privacy should also be allowed. Eating is essentially a public activity in school. Where self-feeding or oral skills are poor, consideration should be given to providing for school lunches foods which the child can manage herself with minimal mess. Some children may cope with sandwiches, others may need soft or mashed foods.

4.3.1 LEARNING IN SCHOOL

During the early school years, the child acquires reading, writing and number skills, which are essential for access into the curriculum. Acquisition of these skills may well be impaired by the disabilities associated with cerebral palsy. Some children with cerebral palsy will have a degree of intellectual impairment, which will affect all aspects of their learning and attainment. Where these learning difficulties are severe, the child may need a developmental curriculum where there is less emphasis on the acquisition of literacy and numeracy skills, and a focus on the development of social and independence skills. Children with moderate degrees of learning difficulty will require a curriculum which is modified to allow for the slower pace of learning and more structured individualized teaching. The learning of children with general intellectual impairment will also be affected by specific perceptual, linguistic and physical difficulties. Recognition of these difficulties, and their potential effects on learning, is just as important in this group of children as it is in children who are of normal intellectual ability.

Attention problems will also affect all aspects of a child's learning in the classroom. Where the child's attention skills are immature, she is likely to have difficulty in integrating visual and auditory aspects of the learning environment. The ability to focus and organize attention appropriately may also be affected by motor, sensory and perceptual difficulties. Some children may not have developed the self-regulation essential to sustained attention. Children who are easily distracted or self-distracting will soon appear to be difficult and perhaps disruptive in a mainstream class.

Where attentional difficulties are severe, individual help from a non-teaching assistant may be necessary if the child is to continue learning alongside others. Most children will not need constant one-to-one supervision, but will require a member of staff to be aware of their difficulties, monitor their performance and facilitate, direct or prompt attention where appropriate. A child's position within the classroom can be planned to maximize auditory and visual inputs and enable easy adult supervision.

(a)   Learning to read

Reading is a complex linguistic skill involving the integration of visual and auditory perception, encoding, sequencing and memory abilities. Nevertheless, most children learn to read without difficulty in their early years at school. An individual child with cerebral palsy may make excellent progress in reading, but as a group, children with cerebral palsy have a substantially increased risk of experiencing reading failure or delay when compared to their non-disabled peers (Rutter *et al.*, 1970; Yule and Rutter, 1970; Segal, 1971; Anderson, 1973).

Associated intellectual impairment will account for some, but not all, of this discrepancy. In the 'Isle of Wight Study' (Rutter *et al.*, 1970), children with cerebral palsy whose intellectual ability was average, showed greater degrees of reading retardation not only in comparison with their non-disabled peers, but also in relation to the attainment of children with equivalent physical disability not attributable to central nervous system damage. This finding led the authors to suggest that specific perceptual and language difficulties may be causative factors in reading difficulty. Children with cerebral palsy have a high incidence of visual perceptual and visual motor difficulties evident on cognitive assessment (Abercrombie, 1964; Wedell, 1973; Cruikshank, 1976), which are clearly likely to affect the process of learning to read, write and spell, but the mechanism of their influence and their interaction with intellectual, physical, social and emotional factors is less well understood.

Reading will also be affected by vision and hearing deficits. Hopefully any sensory difficulties will have been identified well before school entry and, as far as possible, remediated. Where significant difficulties persist, advice and support will be required from appropriate educational specialists. There are, however, some visual difficulties associated with cerebral palsy, such as visual field defects in some children with hemiplegias, and involuntary eye movements in some children with athetoid cerebral palsy, which may significantly affect reading without causing major visual dysfunction in the child's day-to-day life.

In children with severe motor impairment, ease of access to written material may be a factor in early reading. Adult expectations of potential for literacy may be low, particularly for children with expressive communication difficulties. Poor speech intelligibility or absence of spoken communication will also lead to difficulties in determining how well a child is reading and how much she understands of what she reads.

Reading difficulty or delay in a child with cerebral palsy may be multifactorial in cause. In order to develop reading skills optimally the child may need the following.

1. Enhanced access to written material. This will include positioning within the classroom so that she can see the blackboard and other visual aids, the use of a lectern when looking down to table level is difficult, and, where appropriate, a page turner. The introduction of keyboard skills and the use of a microcomputer or typewriter will also provide experiences likely to enhance reading ability (Campbell, 1973). The introduction of a simple strategy such as a ruler to go from line to line may help the child with perceptual difficulties to maintain visual attention to written material.
2. Individual assessment and remediation. To some extent the child with general or specific learning difficulties will have similar needs to a number of other children in mainstream schools. Staff will need information regarding the nature of the child's learning difficulty so that appropriate remedial strategies can be implemented, either individually or in a small group. For children with severe communication difficulties, assessment of reading difficulty and comprehension may require speech therapist and teacher to work together.
3. Parent involvement. With ordinary children who have specific reading retardation, joint working of school and parents has proved effective (Hewson and Tizard, 1980; Topping and Wolfendale, 1985). These approaches should not be ignored with delayed readers who have cerebral palsy, even though the 'organic' basis of their reading deficit tends to receive more emphasis.

(b) Writing

Writing as a means of self-expression is a highly integrative function involving language as well as perceptual and motor processes. Children with cerebral palsy may, because of associated language and intellectual impairment, have difficulty with ideational aspects of writing. Specific deficits in visual and auditory processing may contribute to later spelling difficulties. The most significant way, however, in which cerebral palsy will affect writing is via its impairment of gross and fine motor skills, and associated perceptual–motor deficits.

Motor or perceptual–motor dysfunction will interfere with:

pen/pencil grasp;
application of appropriate pressure;
positional stability;

steadying the paper;
precision and coordination of fine motor movement;
one-to-one correspondence in copying;
copying and reproducing shapes and letters;
use of spacing;
working in horizontal plane;
speed and fluency.

Written work will, as a consequence, be poor in appearance and largely illegible, and yet will have required considerable time and effort. The child will find writing tedious and frustrating. Contrasts between the child's work and that of her peers will be particularly evident. She may be labelled as 'dull' or 'lazy' by teachers, especially when the child's difficulties are due to underlying perceptuo-motor dysfunction rather than to direct effects of her motor impairment.

If the child is not to lose confidence and perhaps abandon attempts at written work, appropriate intervention is essential. This may involve the following.

(i) Attention to positioning   It is important that teachers understand the relationship between posture and graphomotor skills. Many children with cerebral palsy will sit effectively for play by utilizing postures and muscular fixation which enable them to use their upper limbs effectively. This may not be adequate for the degree of precision and intense concentration involved in graphomotor activity. Adaptive seating may range from simple adjustment of height and foot position or use of cushions, through to custom-built or moulded seats. Sometimes the wheelchair will provide the best sitting base in the classroom. In this case the work tray or desk will have to be carefully matched to the child's needs.

(ii) Selection and adaptation of writing tools and materials   Length, weight and shape of barrel (Alston and Hancock, 1986) will be important in the selection of a writing tool for a child. The degree of pressure the child uses will also determine choice of pencil, ballpoint, fibretip, etc. Barrels can be made wider and easier to grip.

The choice of lined paper and the use of tape for securing paper to the table are simple measures which can make the child's tasks significantly easier. With some pupils the use of a simple slant board to replace the horizontal work surface will elicit vastly improved writing.

(iii) Individual tutoring   Specific teaching and remediation of handwriting problems has been found to be valuable for children with spina

bifida (Anderson, 1979) and in children with perceptual motor organization difficulties (Bradley, 1980). An assessment of the child's particular difficulties (Alston and Taylor, 1984; Stott *et al.*, 1985) can form the basis of intervention. The child can be taught and encouraged to practise the movement patterns associated with each letter, beginning and ending at the correct place. Flowing movement patterns and a 'cursive' script will aid fluency and spacing. Where appropriate the child can be encouraged to 'talk' through the movements so that, for example, 'd' would be 'around, right up and down' (Bradley, 1980). Without some specific teaching of correct handwriting skills early on in the school career, the child with cerebral palsy is likely to use inappropriate motor patterns which will be difficult to change later.

(iv) Alternative systems The use of an alternative system of written expression is essential where the child has such severe difficulties that handwriting is not a realistic long-term goal. More commonly the child with cerebral palsy can be enabled to achieve functional handwriting in the future, but may be discouraged and slowed down by her writing. For these children consideration should be given to the use of an alternative system as an adjunct rather than a substitute.

Dictation to a non-teaching assistant who acts as scribe can allow the child creative verbal expression, and help her cope with other aspects of written work in the classroom within the time available. Less expensive is the use of a dictaphone or tape recorder, either for later transcription by the child or others. These approaches require competence in spoken language and may be intrusive within the classroom.

For primary school age children a microcomputer with a simple word processing program will be easier to master and more rewarding in terms of quality of output than a typewriter. Keyboard skills can be introduced early and there are many programs available to help the child to develop keyboard competence. The child with cerebral palsy may still have problems with speed and accuracy of movement when typing. Perceptual difficulties also make it harder for her to monitor and correct her work. A keyguard may minimize typing errors and most children will be motivated to persist in their efforts by the enhanced quality of the work they produce.

Where a child does not have the movement accuracy to use a standard keyboard, other options may be feasible. The child may be able to use an enlarged keyboard with more spacing between the letters, or a single switch or joystick in combination with a keyboard scanning device. Where children use Bliss symbolics, this can be linked in to their written communication system.

One simple adaptation which can be very effective for the child with handwriting difficulty is the use of xeroxed or prepared sheets to replace classroom or workbook copying.

(c)   Number skills

As with literacy, the acquistion of numeracy skills in the child with cerebral palsy will be influenced by intellectual, perceptual and physical factors and by any restriction of learning opportunity and limitation of expectation consequent upon the child's disability. Lewis (1987) notes that arithmetic seems to present even greater problems to children with physical disabilities than reading or writing. School absence appears to be particularly crucial with regard to arithmetical skills (Pringle *et al.*, 1970), perhaps because, unlike reading and writing which, once begun, can be enhanced by independent practice and easily encouraged by parents at home, arithmetical attainment is much more dependent on specific instruction in operation and procedures.

Where a child with cerebral palsy has difficulty in number skills, it will be important to identify relevant cognitive and environmental factors. Most children will require some additional tuition individually or in small groups, employing specific strategies geared towards their learning strengths and needs. School absence will be a particular problem with children who require orthopaedic surgery, where hospital stays and home convalescence may be prolonged. Good liaison with hospital teachers and home tutors will ensure continuity in important core curriculum areas such as arithmetic. In the absence of these services, it may be possible for school and parents to work together to help the child keep up with some aspects of school work. When she returns to school, the child may well need extra help, particularly with arithmetic.

5 *Adolescence*

5.1 Development of self

There is no definite time for the onset of puberty, nor can a definite age be stated by which the passage through adolescence has been completed. For the purpose of this chapter the adolescent period will cover the years between 10 and 16. The ease with which the adolescent copes with this period is dependent upon how successful he has been as a child in mastering the earlier stages of development. Some may enjoy their emerging self-awareness, while others find the combination of physical and emotional changes a bewildering experience.

During puberty growth is accelerated, starting earlier in girls than in boys, and the body changes in shape to show the characteristic male or female appearance. Muscle strength and coordination improve so that, during late adolescence, physical fitness and athletic prowess will often reach a peak. It is also a time when the young are ready for new ideas.

Sexual maturity is accompanied by an increased awareness of one's own as well as others' sexuality. It is a time for organizing behaviour that is acceptable to the individual and to society at large.

The adolescent becomes subject to peer pressure and the influence of the media. He is more aware of the way in which his family behave, what his parents are like as individuals, and the circumstances in which they make a living. Our society continues to become increasingly complex, with such issues as race, unemployment, marital disharmony and the conflicting arguments about what is moral behaviour. The adolescent is faced with the dilemma of matching his ideals with the realities of society.

The adolescent should receive parental encouragement to accept responsibility for personal actions and for decisions as to what is reasonable behaviour. It is a time for risk-taking and challenge, with mood swings from excitement to misery, but with adult cooperation and understanding the majority of adolescents will start adult life with confidence and hope.

5.1.1   IMPACT OF CEREBRAL PALSY ON THE ADOLESCENT

The period of early adolescence is an appropriate time for a reappraisal of health status and needs: a review of the progress made so far, the skills which have emerged and the learning opportunities and support that will be needed to overcome the disability.

(a)   Understanding the condition

It is easy to assume that a disabled adolescent understands his or her physical condition, but this may not always be the case. A survey carried out in 1982 by Madge and Fassam entitled 'Ask the Children' found that physically disabled children were often uninformed about their own condition and adults had not discussed this with them. Most children when questioned welcomed the opportunity to talk about their disability.

Parents and teachers in particular need to pick up on questions at the time the adolescent initiates them because this is a delicate area, and one which it can be painful to discuss. Freeman (1970) writes that 'Not telling the patient the truth about his handicap and the procedures associated with its management may have been the policy during childhood, but the teenager usually needs fresh understanding and an opportunity to discuss his feelings and fears for the future in the light of his changed awareness of himself.'

When talking to a young person about cerebral palsy, it needs to be explained that the condition is not a specific diagnosis but a name given to a range of disabilities resulting from damage to the brain and central nervous system. This may help them to understand that the symptoms vary in severity, in case they have fears that their condition may deteriorate or be hereditary. They may also need to reconsider previously held hopes that one day they will be cured. Minde's study in 1978 found that, between the ages of 10 and 14 years, adolescents with cerebral palsy (and their parents) developed increased awareness of the permanence of their handicap.

At times decisions need to be made about orthopaedic intervention or cosmetic surgery, and it is appropriate that these be shared with the young person as involvement in making choices is a useful preparation for adulthood. Parents will have to decide at what stage the adolescent is sufficiently mature to be given this responsibility and this may sometimes mean deferring treatment until the young person can make an informed decision.

(b)   Body matters

Physical changes at the onset of puberty are at the forefront of the adolescent's daily living experiences. Fear or embarrassment may prevent the adolescent from approaching adults and peers to get reassurance and leave him trying to make sense of these changes for himself. He has to find ways of understanding that his changing appearance is not something to be frightened about. For girls, bodily changes affect their appearance more noticeably with the development of breasts. For boys, the development of their genitalia is outwardly less apparent but equally anxiety provoking in terms of comparisons or fantasies about what should be happening. It may come as a relief to realize that, in their attitudes towards sexual development, the adolescent with cerebral palsy is the same as his peers.

Adolescents start to find out intuitively the pleasurable experience that masturbation can bring. For girls, the onset of menstruation is a major issue and the management of periods in terms of hygiene can present practical difficulties as well as discomfort and pain.

Parents should have a positive role to play during this developmental phase by providing opportunities for discussion with their children. They may, however, need encouragement from professionals to tackle this sensitive issue and the provision of specialized literature can be of help. Some parents, however, could find the task too difficult and school staff/counsellors should be available for consultation. It has to be remembered that a physical disability affecting mobility may prevent the adolescent from obtaining his own information about sex and birth control.

Bodily self-examination and experimentation may be restricted by a physical handicap and lack of privacy. Bax and Oswin (1967) commented that whereas the normal adolescent can get away from prying eyes to experiment, the adolescent with cerebral palsy is likely to be closely supervised and may have little, if any, privacy. Parents can help by creating opportunities at appropriate times, e.g. bathing. Those who also have intellectual impairment have the same needs as any young person, but have to be taught that sexual activity is only acceptable in private.

Alongside the awakening of sexuality comes a period of increased growth that can make the adolescent gangly and awkward – more so if he has minimal control over his bodily movements. These inescapable changes in the adolescent's appearance lead him into issues of how he is going to handle this emerging person in his social environment.

(c) Opportunities for self-expression

Greater pressures come to bear on children as they move into adolescence and become more aware of themselves in relation to their peers. They may experience themselves as a disappointment and their adjustment will be influenced by parental and peer acceptance. For some, determination and a sense of humour can bring increased physical control over the mild hemiplegia or diplegia. For others the need to join their peers will persuade them to use wheelchairs to give them a new independence. Darling and Darling (1982) confirmed that high self-esteem is an important index of adjustment.

Bodily changes bring opportunities to experiment with one's personal appearance. The adolescent becomes a target for the mass media and advertising world to influence and even exploit. Trends are short-lived but feed into the adolescent's excitement at this period of change. No longer is he an offshoot of his parents, but an individual developing his own likes and dislikes and desperately wanting to exercise his own choices in respect of spending pocket money and choosing his own clothes and hairstyle. In general, by mid-adolescence, the young person should be expected by his parents to take some responsibility in managing small sums of money. The awareness of money values and the ability to budget is a desirable skill that needs to be acquired. Most adolescents will learn through managing their pocket money. This is equally applicable to the adolescent with a physical disability, who may, in the United Kingdom, become entitled to state benefits in his own right at 16 years of age.

Opportunities for self-expression will be restricted by the physical limitations placed on the adolescent with cerebral palsy, who is dependent on others for outings. Where possible, parents and carers should involve them in shopping trips to choose their own purchases. In this way parents can help to alleviate the frustration of the adolescent by involving him in personal decisions and thereby preparing him for adult life.

Some parents may be reluctant to relinquish control over their child at a time when they still have to attend to many of his personal needs. This prolonged state of dependency creates a dilemma for parent and child alike, and some young people will never achieve the desired state of autonomy. Greengross (1980) describes this interdependency as follows:

> Boundaries are impossible to define, for physical dependency and emotional control are inextricably mixed; and parents find themselves both involved and influential in the decisions that their children are making: and their children cannot be free. They cannot let their children go and this is as damaging to the parent as it is to the child.

(d) Personal adjustment

From the relative security of his home base, the adolescent challenges his parents, school and society at large in the search for a sense of identity. The timing and intensity varies from individual to individual: some adolescents begin to question parental decisions, lose their temper in frustration, or rebel in more destructive ways.

However, some adolescents with cerebral palsy have the unenviable task of expressing their inner turmoil hampered by poor communication skills and restricted mobility. They may be unable to argue, walk out of the room, slam doors, or stay for hours in bed. Their attempts at rebellion, therefore, may have to be non-verbal, visual, and by means of non-cooperation. In addition, because these young people are dependent on their parents for physical care, it may not be easy for them to challenge parental values that could in turn threaten their own security.

If the adolescent with cerebral palsy has not gained full control of his body in his pre-pubertal phase, the additional loss of control brought about by his sexual development and growth spurt may add to feelings of helplessness. Self-confidence and self-esteem can easily be undermined during this period and the young person's self-worth put in question.

Sensitivity, vulnerability and frustration may reveal themselves in anger, withdrawal, depression and lethargy. The adolescent needs to find acceptable ways of expressing these feelings, vividly described here by one young adolescent: 'I felt lonely and restless . . . all the friendly ties that I had formed in my childhood were broken by the rift that adolescence had wrought between myself and the boys I had played with as a child . . . instead of coming to a better understanding of my handicap as I got older, I only became more troubled and bitter.' Originally set down in 1954 – by Christy Brown in *My Left Foot* – such feelings are echoed by successive generations and are just as relevant in today's world.

The observations of child care staff at a local respite unit for physically handicapped children and adolescents very much confirm the turmoil and uncertainty experienced by the developing youngster. The staff find that the generally positive self-image of the younger child gives way to a negative one as adolescence advances; with an increasing awareness of life's realities comes a rising despondency. There are expectations upon the adolescent of greater self-reliance and he feels himself to be in competition *vis à vis* more able-bodied peers. Contact with school friends often diminishes. There is the problem of finding a partner and growing fears concerning the mortality of parents. The troubled feelings stemming from these pressures manifest themselves periodically in anger, lethargy, depression, increased dependency, and references to suicide. The staff felt that this ultimately led to a demoralizing acceptance of the situation by their young charges.

It is important for parents and involved professionals to be aware of such issues that trouble the teenager's mind, for if these are not acknowledged, they may remain unresolved. Professionals may need or prefer at times to look at these issues by working with the adolescent's parents. They should be aware, however, that this approach may only prolong the adolescent's dependency.

The adolescent with cerebral palsy, like any other young person, should be given opportunities by professionals to express himself in his own right. He may not want to share 'secret' intimate feelings with close family members and his wish for counselling from an impartial outsider should be respected. In this way, the adolescent can be encouraged to state his own views directly and lessen the dependency on adults to communicate for him. He will gain confidence and self-esteem from knowing that he is respected and valued as an individual, with his own thoughts and feelings.

5.2   Moving towards personal independence

The personal needs of the child have, perhaps unquestioningly, been met by the parents and other people in contact with the child. Now the parents are beginning to see that their child is developing into a young adult. They may realize that the child should have greater privacy and independence in attending to personal care, but do not see how they, the parents, can alter the habits ingrained and developed over several years. Cooperation with professionals may be needed in order to make progress in this area, and ideally the adolescent, parents, paramedical and teaching staff can all work together as a team.

The young handicapped person needs to develop a positive attitude towards his abilities in order to learn how to manage personal care tasks and daily living activities. Such teaching can be incorporated into a school curriculum in such a way that the adolescent is able to work and progress at his own level of physical and emotional ability. The aims of the teaching programme are to assess and develop the adolescent's physical status and functional abilities in managing personal and household skills. Individuals will each need to be helped to organize themselves in their own environment and it is vital that the professionals involved make a realistic assessment: too high an expectation on the adolescent can create feelings of failure and mistrust, which in turn lead to a loss of self-confidence. To avoid this, the adolescent must be encouraged to see himself as actively rather than passively involved in attaining the objectives and his feelings acknowledged. He also needs to have motivation and to be rewarded by some degree of success. The goals themselves can be simple or complex, ranging from physically managing to remove socks to transferring independently into and out of a car.

Before drawing up a programme, the therapist needs to visit home to assess the adolescent's functional ability in the home environment, which may lack some of the facilities available in a school. Objectives can then be discussed and agreed with parents. In working with the family, the therapist should be perceptive to the needs of other family members, and how this affects the management of the child. Different cultural and religious backgrounds will have a bearing on the family's expectations of their child and the manner in which tasks are completed. The therapist needs, therefore, to gain an understanding of the family's attitudes and adapt the teaching programme accordingly.

Each aspect of personal care will have to be broken down to achievable stages and individual tasks worked at until the adolescent can complete the activity to the best of his ability. The adolescent works on the individual skills and then learns how to sequence them together, as illustrated in the following example – a bedtime routine for a girl of 14 years who has spastic quadriplegia and uses a powered wheelchair at school and a rollator at home.

Undressing	→ Discuss what is most suitable clothing, that is:
Sitting on chair	1. physically managable;
Top half	2. attractive/fashionable and still appropriate;
Bottom half	3. how to choose what to wear and what to say;
Socks and shoes	4. methods of buying, e.g. catalogues or shops.

Toiletting	→ Obstacle courses incorporating general mobility of walking and rolling, transferring to and from different heights, practising different movements required in removal of clothing, bedding, etc. in games.
From rollator (used at home)	
From wheelchair (used at school)	
Move to toilet	
Remove lower clothing	
Transfer on to toilet	→ Preparation activities with small goals, e.g. undressing/dressing lower clothing:
Clean self	
Manage clothing	1. standing and holding with one hand only;
Transfer off toilet	2. transfers.

Clean teeth	
Take cap off toothpaste	→ Discussion of teeth care, how to do it effectively and why. It is unpleasant for self and others not to clean teeth. How frequently do you brush teeth and visit dentist?
Put toothpaste on brush	
Clean teeth	→ Best position to clean teeth.
Rinse out mouth	→ Discuss types of toothpaste dispensers and brushes.

Bathing	
Move to edge of bath on rollator or wheelchair	→ Discussion on personal hygiene, why, how frequently should you wash. What areas do you take special care over. What are the difficulties and how do you overcome them?
Transfer to bath seat in bath	→ Discussion and practical demonstration on regulating temperature of bath water.
Lower into bath	→ Safety factors of hot water and wet and slippery surfaces.
Lift up on to bath seat	→ Obstacle courses incorporating general mobility of walking, rolling, transferring.
Transfer out of bath	

Getting into bed	
Move to bed	→ Discuss and try different types of bedding, height of beds, and softness of mattress.
Move back bedding and transfer on to bed	
Shift down bed into comfortable position	
Pull bedding up over self	

Such programmes are obviously time-consuming and difficult for busy parents to undertake at home. It is, therefore, more realistic for the initial work to be practised in school and reinforced by carers at home. Where progress is painstaking, there is the temptation to complete tasks for the disabled person to save time and avoid frustration. Time and patience are needed by all parties concerned if the young person is to be helped to master these new skills.

One approach to teaching self-help skills is to work with small groups of approximately five young people of the same sex. The group can create an atmosphere of trust, empathy and encouragement, which helps to develop personal confidence, motivation and self-worth. It can help to develop an awareness of the personal problems of others as well as one's own, which leads to mutual sharing, offering advice, and praise. The peer group are also quick to comment on inappropriate behaviour from another member and this can be more effective than adult correction. Goals which are difficult to achieve or embarrassing to discuss can sometimes be broached more easily in a group situation than with an individual. This is because the material is less threatening when the problem is discussed in general terms rather than focusing on one person. It is important to remember that learning can be fun, and this is an aspect which can be fostered in a group situation.

The adolescent should be encouraged to see the funny side of a mishap rather than viewing this as a failure. Sharing these experiences within the group may help the adolescent's adjustment to his disability.

Alongside the acquisition of self-help skills, the disabled adolescent needs to learn 'social' or 'life-skills' that will effectively equip him to handle daily living situations and relationships in the world outside his family and school. It can be equally effective to consider teaching such social skills within a group situation, perhaps at school or in a youth club. It is probable that physical difficulties will restrict the opportunities the adolescent with cerebral palsy has for personal decision making and problem solving. Within the safety of a small group the adolescent can be given opportunities to practise the skills that will help him feel he has some degree of control over decisions and choices that affect his daily life.

Bell and Quintal (1985) describe a Life Skills Programme that was set up for physically disabled adolescents in a formalized group. Participants found it a satisfactory and positive way of looking at the issues facing them in their search for independence. An important aspect was the experience of contact with positive role models and the opportunity to develop a sense of self-esteem. It became evident that 'a strong sense of self-esteem is one of the most valuable resources any adolescent can possess'.

If the young person with cerebral palsy can be given opportunities to gain confidence in areas of personal and social competence whilst still an adolescent, his sense of well-being can be enhanced. He will be encouraged to develop effective coping mechanisms and adaptive responses to situations he is likely to encounter as he enters adulthood. This may prepare him to take more initiative to put the able-bodied at their ease and thus help them to develop a more realistic understanding of what it is like to be disabled.

5.3   The transfer from family group to peer group

Adolescence is the time to move away from the intensity of family relationships and to seek out an identity within the peer group. It may not be an individual but a collective identity that emerges initially, as the means of gaining security and acceptance. This prepares the way to moving on to greater individuation later on in adolescence. The process of gradual separation from the family group is more complicated for the handicapped adolescent because of problems of mobility and social acceptance. He will want to mix more with friends and concentrate on hobbies and leisure interests that are not shared with parents. Attendance at a special school can be isolating because school friends are unlikely to live nearby. Those at mainstream school may find themselves unable to keep pace with their physically more agile peers. Youth clubs catering for able-bodied and disabled youngsters together may be one way of experiencing heterosexual relationships.

School plays an important role in broadening the adolescent's horizons beyond the immediate family circle and neighbourhood network. It introduces new opportunities for outside activities that the adolescent may wish to take advantage of, such as youth clubs, swimming and holidays away from home. School can thus legitimize the break away from the family for the adolescent by making it socially acceptable and by sharing in the risks of letting go. Fear of rejection or failure may inhibit efforts to establish relationships and try new ventures, but risks must be taken if social competence is to be achieved.

Madge and Fassam (1982) concluded that 'Senior pupils in special education were becoming more reliant on their parents for social outings at a time when able-bodied adolescents were beginning to break their ties with home by spending more time with friends and establishing an independent life'.

Access to a means of transport will be necessary for the more seriously disabled to participate in social activities. Financial help to provide transport is sometimes available through statutory allowances or voluntary bodies. For some the opportunities for recreation are so limited that it is encumbent upon service providers to recognize and meet the needs of the adolescent so that these youngsters do not have to compromise and experience the outside world at one remove through television, magazines or via siblings.

5.3.1   AN ADOLESCENT'S VIEWPOINT

In this chapter we have attempted to outline the general issues relevant to the young adolescent with cerebral palsy. The following extract is taken from an interview carried out by a Ryegate member of staff with an adolescent girl, 'K', aged 16 years, who has ataxic cerebral palsy and dystonia. She attends a special unit attached to an ordinary school and is of normal intelligence. It is hoped that this will give a personal insight into the impact of cerebral palsy for the adolescent.

Q: What disorder do you think you have and how do you explain it to others?

A: Cerebral palsy, and it is because I was short of oxygen when I was born. I was a breech delivery and the cord was damaged.

Q: Do people ask you for more details?

A: Yes. They ask what I can do and I tell them that I can do quite a lot because I am getting better at doing things, but I am not sure whether I am just getting better or coping better because I am older. Some teachers ask what I can do, others always offer help. Some assume you cannot do things, so I wait until I know them better and then I ask if I can do things myself, for example, putting paper into the typewriter. Most days I can do it by myself, but there are some days which are better than others and on difficult days I recognize that time is being wasted, and so then I want to ask for help. I am worse if I am nervous or apprehensive about exams.

Q: Do you belong to any club or organization?

A: Yes. I go to youth club every Friday at the local church. Dad takes both of us [she has a sister]. I don't go out alone.

Q: Have you been on any holidays away from your parents?

A: Yes. I went with the club to London. Mother was worried sick but we enjoyed it.

Q: Do you go swimming?

A: Well, I can swim and I enjoy swimming, but I do not enjoy going to the baths because I do not like getting out of the water, drying and dressing myself. It's the thought of all the trouble.

Q: Do you think your family is pleased with you and your progress?

A: Yes, very pleased. Both my parents give me encouragement. My mother has always encouraged me to do as much as possible.

Q: Do you feel, as most people do, unhappy or sad or lonely at times?

A: Well, on the whole I am a happy sort of person, no more sad or lonely than the average. I like to have a moan, occasionally a cry, but I will talk in a sick joke sort of way with my sister and then we can have a laugh.

Q: Remembering the quarrels you had with your mother when you were around 12 and 13, what do you feel caused these?

A: Well, it's easier now. I think I was frustrated and angry about my problems when I was younger, but I think it was normal adolescence. I quarrel less with my sister. We have the same sense of humour.

Q: Do you resent being helped?

A: Mother is worried about me spilling things and when she watches me she will stop me from pouring hot liquids because I am spilling it into the saucer or on to the table top, but at school I try and I just make a mess and wipe it up afterwards.

Q: Do you think you would like to live away from home?

A: Well, I think that if I left home I would be lonely. I would also have difficulty with washing my hair and cutting my nails, but I could go to a hairdresser and have my nails done there. I still have to ask my mother to do some things like this, including shaving under my arms which is impossible. We are looking for ways around problems.

Q: Do you think you will have children?

A: No, I don't think I will have a baby. I am not interested in babies or little children. I don't think I have the patience and I think I would find it difficult. What I want is a good job and a husband with a good job and a high standard of living. I need to be able to pay someone to look after us, like nannies, a cook or housekeeper. You know, like the Royal Family!

5.4   Family issues

For parents, their children's progression into adolescence signifies a time when they themselves will have more freedom and be less tied to the physical care of their offspring. This expectation may never be realized for those whose child has a significant disability and this can produce conflicting feelings. As parents are getting older they are less able to deal with the physical and emotional demands made on them when their own health is no longer assured. There may be the added complication of ageing grandparents, who have been able to help out in the past, and who now need more care themselves.

Many parents have fears about what will happen to their child if they die and need to be looking toward future resources both inside and outside the family. Siblings may have had a role in the family as carers and are now needing to make their own lives. There may be pressures on them to take the responsibility for their handicapped brother or sister and they may have guilt feelings about spending less time at home. Likewise, for younger siblings, the restrictions on family outings and social activities because of the handicapped member can be a source of resentment. Discussion about these issues in the family can relieve tensions which arise, but the problem highlights the need to seek outside support, such as respite care facilities.

The introduction of respite care can occur before adolescence but becomes more pressing as the parents get older. This can involve a residential setting or a family placement, depending on the services available and individual preference. Parents sometimes need to adjust to the idea of relinquishing the care of their child to someone else and this can be the beginning of the gradual process of 'letting go'. Counselling may be needed to help parents cope with any feelings of guilt that arise because they are having to call on outside services to look after their son or daughter. If reassurance can be given that they are not failing as parents, it can ease their anxieties and help them view the services in a more positive light. Respite care can also be a way in which the adolescent develops friendships independent of the family and the residential setting offers opportunities for mixing in a peer group.

The natural instinct for parents is to want to protect their offspring and shield them from potentially hurtful situations. Handicapped adolescents may be perceived as more vulnerable than their able-bodied peers and parents can become overprotective. This will prevent the adolescent from being able to try out new situations which lead to success or failure. Risk-taking is nevertheless a part of the maturation process and one through which we become aware of our strengths and weaknesses. Thus, for some adolescents, time away from home may be the only opportunity for developing a sense of independence.

There are practical ways in which greater independence can be achieved in the home by the provision of aids that will allow the adolescent to attend to his own personal needs, for example, toilet aids or the provision of a shower. Adaptations to the home, such as door widening or downstairs facilities, can increase indoor mobility for those in a wheelchair. Where the young person is more highly dependent, the provision of appropriate equipment for lifting may be one of the factors that determines whether parents can continue as carers. There is specialist advice available on housing matters and parents may need guidance on the options available. Even though the house itself may not be suitable for major adaptations, minor alterations can improve the quality of life for the whole family. In particular, the adolescent's need for privacy has to be borne in mind. Ideally, the provision of separate facilities should be considered, but failing this, members of the family can be encouraged to allow the handicapped adolescent privacy for personal hygiene.

Family attitudes and cultural expectations will inevitably influence the young person's adjustment to adolescence and to his disability. Outside agencies such as schools and social services should ideally be in partnership with parents helping the young person to achieve a degree of independence that is realistic to his physical capability. All have a role to play in enabling the adolescent to make the transition into adulthood.

5.4.1 ADJUSTMENT TO SOCIETAL NORMS

Few people have direct experience of disability and the majority do not think to question existing attitudes that are prejudicial. The young person with cerebral palsy will encounter a variety of unpredictable reactions from members of the public that can range from caring concern to hostile avoidance. The public's discomfort in the presence of a handicapped person produces insensitive responses that arise from a lack of understanding about the disability. Some of the physical effects of cerebral palsy, such as uncontrolled body movements, dribbling and speech difficulties, can be mistakenly assumed to indicate limited intellectual abilities. There is, therefore, a tendency to see the disability before the person and this creates a barrier that needs to be overcome if relationships are to be formed.

The extent to which a handicapped person can be integrated into society depends on the tolerance and understanding shown towards them by the able-bodied. Concepts such as normalization may have been accepted by professionals but are still far from being put into practice at a public or individual level. For the adolescent with cerebral palsy the wish to belong and to be accepted as an equal may exist but never be realized. The move away from the family environment exposes the young person to a mixture of public attitudes and expectations. Society appears to demand more of its weaker members in terms of their adjustment than it does of its able-bodied members. It is the disabled person who has to find ways of fitting in with the lifestyle of a competitive and mobile society, and few compromises are made to accommodate the needs of the disabled.

Loring and Burn (1975) comment that the handicapped child has to learn not only to accept the limitations placed upon him by his handicap, but also how to measure up to all the demands which society places upon him. 'Very often his task is made even more difficult by the preconceived notions that society itself has of the handicapped, and the handicapped person then finds himself in a situation in society in which he has to prove himself in his own right as an ordinary human being.'

The education of the public is a slow process but can be influenced by government policies and legislation. For example, measures can be taken to improve access to public places for wheelchair users and this creates a physical environment in which the presence of handicapped people is acknowledged. Voluntary bodies and self-help organizations can act as pressure groups and promote publicity to raise the general level of understanding of the public concerning the difficulties faced by the disabled.

The media could also play a more active role to inform and re-educate the general public in order to promote awareness of the needs and rights of disabled people in our society. Rarely are the successes of the disabled considered newsworthy, whether in the field of sport or entertainment, or in the arts. By portraying the disabled as ordinary people who are in most respects the same as everyone else and similarly capable of outstanding achievement, the media would allow the adolescent with a disability the chance to develop a positive self-image.

6 *The young adult*

Unlike adolescence, the start of adulthood is not marked by any major physical changes. Legally in Britain young people may marry at 16 and start their own families. However, they are not able to drive a car before 17, neither vote nor buy alcoholic drinks until 18, nor can they be sent to prison before 21. At 18 some young people will still be in full-time education, financially supported by their parents. Others will be gainfully employed in the working world and perhaps be living away from the family, either on their own or with other young people. Some may have already begun a family of their own. Some, however, will already have joined the ranks of the long-term unemployed, living on state benefits which may be inadequate.

It is perhaps easier to define adulthood by looking at the tasks to be performed and at the expectations that society has of young adults. In developed 'Western society' the achievement of adult status usually includes having some form of occupation after schooling and secondly gaining personal independence in various spheres of life. There is an expectation of a gradual decreasing dependency on the family, and a transition to a new family system, sometimes a complete role reversal when parents become dependent on their children. If young adults remain in their own homes they will probably be expected to make a financial contribution to the household. Parents will have decreasing authority over their personal and sexual relationships, and no legal authority to make decisions or plan courses of action for them to follow – how a young person chooses to spend her leisure time can no longer be controlled by her parents. Society expects the young adult to be in control of her personal world, to take responsibility for her actions, and to begin to contribute to the well-being of the community. Young adulthood is the time when people need to be establishing their role in the community in order to achieve self-respect and to gain acceptance not only from their peer group but also the larger community in which they function. It is a time when choices have to be made and expectations and personal goals come to be tested, perhaps for the first time.

For young people with cerebral palsy there are many hurdles to be overcome before 'adulthood' (as described above) can be reached. The degree of difficulty will obviously be affected by the severity of the impairment. However, equally important are two further aspects, firstly how the young person's childhood and general upbringing have helped her to understand and live with her impairment. 'One of the most difficult things throughout my childhood was really finding out who I was and what I was because my whole identity as a person was defined as a CP. It was really a long time before I felt I had a name and an identity other than by disability' (Richardson, 1972). The second, and more important aspect, is how society views and accommodates persons with disabilities.

> To be disabled in the community is to be a second class member of it . . . In the past disabled people became accustomed to being outcasts, disempowered. In a word, disabled people were oppressed. Oppression is the systematic mistreatment of one group by another. For us this is the way in which society assumes everyone is able-bodied. So we end up with buildings we can't get into, with jobs designed so that we can't work in them. (Roberts, 1985)

How do these three factors affect the tasks to be achieved by the young person with cerebral palsy in order to reach adulthood? The tasks can be divided into four main areas:

1. occupation after schooling;
2. achieving personal autonomy and independence;
3. changing family patterns and establishing adult personal relationships;
4. establishing a role and participating in the larger community.

6.1   Occupation after schooling

In Britain a young person will normally leave school between the ages of 16 and 18. There are various options after this – further education in a university or college, going into a youth training scheme, finding a job in the open market, or becoming unemployed. For those with disabilities there are also sheltered placement schemes, adult training centres and various day centres. The choice is usually made by looking at the young people's scholastic records, the wishes of the young people themselves, and their family, and linking these up with the opportunities available – often with the help of the Careers Service.

The young person with cerebral palsy has difficulties in all three areas. Many will have been in special schools, and although able to stay on an extra year, many will leave with no externally recognized qualifications and with a much lower standard of educational achievement than most leaving from a mainstream school. The reasons for this are varied – for example, time off school due to hospitalization, the nature of the school curriculum including physiotherapy and activities of daily living, the learning difficulties of the young person – but for whatever reason, these young people are therefore at a disadvantage compared to their able-bodied peers when competing for further training and jobs.

How do young people decide what they are interested in? Often they model themselves on a member of the family, a media personality, or other significant people in their life. For young people with disabilities there are very limited positive role models available, especially with so much emphasis on the 'healthy perfect body'. Occupations carried out by other members of the family may not seem achievable. Young people at special schools will have friends with similar problems, which often leads to unrealistic or low expectations.

> As the study progressed, interviewers gained the impression that many of the young interviewees had very poor self-esteem and rather low expectations from life. Although some of the control group too are depressed about unemployment and worried about the future, many of the young adults in the survey seem to lack a strong self-image and sense of personal worth and importance. (Royal Devon and Exeter Hospital, 1985)

Parents may also have come to accept very low expectations for their disabled children. It is at this time that information about the possibilities open to young people is vital and professionals involved with young people must help them to obtain as much information as possible if they are to have any real choice. Over the past few years in Britain there have been great steps taken by different disability groups – for example, Centres for Integrated/Independent Living and DIAL (Disability Information Advice Line) – to provide better information and advice to people with disabilities.

The able-bodied young person, armed with ambitions, qualifications and knowledge of opportunities, is left to pursue whatever course is open to her. For the young person with disability there is perhaps another hurdle to overcome – 'the professional assessment of her capabilities'. Assessment is a strong political weapon. While on one hand it can be seen as helping the individual to assess his own capabilities and needs, on the other hand it can be seen as a method of prolonging the dependency role, acting as a barrier to resources, and lastly as siting disability exclusively in the individual. The need for assessment can be seen as the previous failure of services to equip the individual to assess her own needs. Assessment will be mentioned in more detail in the next section, when discussing autonomy and independence, but narrowly confined to occupation, it can be seen to be of little help. Rather, perhaps, it should be the jobs that are assessed to see how they can be changed to accommodate disability. In Britain and other countries in Europe several successes have been recorded of people with disabilities doing jobs which previously would not have seemed possible. In the past certain jobs have been reserved for the disabled – usually the unskilled and low paid – but the trend is now for many jobs to be accessible to persons with disabilities. Initial help and grants from government to employers are now available to alter the physical environment of work sites to help make this possible.

Rather depressingly, however, a recent survey puts into sharp focus what the occupations of young people with disabilities are.

> The findings of this study underline the limited opportunities for young people with disabilities in further education and employment training, their dependence on day care and the difficulties they face in finding paid employment . . . there are three implications. First the vast majority of young people with disabilities in the sample can look forward to an occupational role which is both undervalued by and segregated from ordinary adult society. Secondly, they face long term dependence on the social security system, incomes close to the official poverty line and low living standards. Thirdly, and as a consequence, they will have few opportunities to develop control and responsibility for their own lives. (Hirst, 1987)

Often further education has to be in special colleges because of difficult physical access to mainstream universities and college. The opportunities open to the young person at the end of these courses may not be greatly increased and, as mentioned by Hirst above, the occupation available may be in day centre placements. In many parts of Britain the day centres are provided to cater for all people with disability and because of the increase of disability with age, these centres are mainly used by the elderly. In some areas there are special day centres for young people with disabilities and, although an improvement, they again provide a segregated environment which can foster low expectations and high dependency.

Some young people with cerebral palsy are so severely disabled that they 'need help to explore the opportunities for developing themselves as people and gaining skills through alternatives. Perhaps by looking at the implications of unemployment for non-disabled young people and what alternatives they have, joint ideas might be developed' (Twitchin, 1981). So often, however, mobility and access problems lead to segregation, and because of segregation in school years, mixing young people with disabilities and those without has to be in contrived settings when often the helper/disabled model is unwittingly reinforced.

People with disabilities have limited opportunities to establish self-esteem and a role in the community. Employment may be one of the few opportunities for this to take place and it is crucial, therefore, that all efforts should be made to help young people with cerebral palsy to find an occupation.

> Despite the spreading rumour that the traditional 'work ethic' of western societies is rapidly declining, the significance of work as the major proof of adult status and active participation in society remains uncontested. The work one does not only defines one's place in society, it determines largely the material quality of life, but also impinges upon one's sense of competence and self esteem. (CERI/OECD, 1987)

The paper from which the above is taken goes on to state that work provides a personal identity, an opportunity to contribute to society, widens social contact, gives structure to a day and is further education and training in itself. All these are as crucial to young people with disabilities as their able-bodied peers.

6.2   Achieving personal autonomy and independence

What does personal independence and autonomy mean? No one in present day Western society is totally independent – we all need services and resources from other people. Independence is often construed in terms of physical tasks which can be performed unaided. An alternative perspective, however, is to consider the individual's autonomy in making personal and economic decisions and the quality of life which can be experienced given adequate help.

First and foremost, all young people need somewhere to live, and young adulthood is often the time when the break is made away from 'home'. Parents/carers in differing degree may help or put up resistance to ideas of moving away, but in addition, young people with disabilities will also need/have to consult the 'caring professions' if extra resources are required. Traditionally people with disabilities have been seen to need some sort of 'care', either in institutions/homes or through remaining with their parents. Now, with 'moves into the community', more young people with disabilities are looking into the possibility of living on their own, and centres for independent/ integrated living are growing up to provide help and information to enable them to do so.

Suitable housing needs to be available,

> Yet the concept of special needs is wholly misleading. The needs of people with disability in terms of housing are no different from the population at large. There is no model for disabled persons' housing that will appeal to everyone and we believe that the first requirements must be a plea for choice and a variety of provision in both public and private sector accommodation. This may include warden supervised and communal dwellings, but it is important that such 'service-rich' accommodation should be recognised and regarded as only part of a much broader range of options.

If housing needs are to be met wherever they occur, rather than in clusters of disabled housing, then other services, e.g. home helps, family aides, personal care assistants and district nurses, have to be delivered in a flexible way. This is often seen as a stumbling block, but the benefits that accrue from this may well outweigh the problems; the young people can stay near family and friends in a community they know, the housing is not easily recognizable as disabled housing, and hence not such an easy target for vandalism, and there is securer tenancy for anyone living with a person with a disability.

Another area where personal autonomy needs to be aimed for is in the care and control of the young person's body – in the activities of daily living, e.g. toiletting and personal hygiene, cooking, learning to recognize signs of ill health, and taking responsibility for their bodies.

> The progress of a child's development . . . mostly stops at a disappointing level . . . the adolescent child often fails to assume the responsibility appropriate to his age and fails to acquire the activities of daily living. This may be the result of 'shared parenthood'. The young person's body seems 'strange', almost public property. The child remains dependent upon its parents for complete care. We conclude that 'shared parenthood' of the 'child of science' has obstructed its path to adulthood. (Scheers *et al.*, 1984)

Though this quotation is in relation to young people with spina bifida, the same protective paediatric service is given to children with cerebral palsy, with often the same results.

A more gradual fading out of paediatric care into an accessible adult point of reference would seem to be called for. Over the past few years there has been much reference made to the 'cliff phenomenon', where young people with disabilities at the age of around 16 move from protective care into the adult world where few services exist. This has led to demand for 'cradle to grave services' for people with disabilities and a massive expansion of adult disability provision as called for in *Physical Disability in 1986 and Beyond* (Royal College of Physicians, 1986). Many services provided or demanded at the moment are remedial, in that they are rectifying the failure of earlier services – e.g. calls for 'independence training units'. Independence and autonomy has to be based on solid foundations encouraged throughout the young person's childhood by both family and the professionals. Parents have to learn to let their now grown-up children take responsibility for their actions, which often means taking risks. However, there are medical/paramedical services that are needed by the young person with cerebral palsy that will not be needed by their able-bodied peers, e.g. there may be problems with incontinence, with care of pressure sores, a need for physiotherapy, and advice. These services must be provided in the most acceptable way to the young people and with easy accessibility.

Assessment was mentioned earlier in terms of occupational assessment. Assessment can be of great use when looking at the activities of daily living in considering new ways to overcome disability and by professionals offering as much information as possible for the disabled person from which to make informed choices. However, it must always be remembered that the needs perceived in assessment are perceived by the young person, the family, and the professionals, and not merely imposed by the professionals. In Britain, these professionals are often the route to the service providers and so can greatly affect the quality of life of young people with disabilities, a quality that is very much affected by the services available. A recent Act of Parliament in Britain has placed a legal responsibility on local authorities to assess the needs of people with disabilities, and their carers, and to provide the services identified. (HMSO, 1986).

It is the parents and young people themselves who are usually the experts by the time the person with disability reaches adulthood. 'Carers' can often be irritated by lack of knowledge on the part of certain 'professionals'. Easily accessible information is needed for professionals as well as their clients and more flow of information between professionals. Many staff who work with adults have little training in the area of disability and must be prepared to listen carefully to their clients. Staff in day centres have been trained to 'care' which may well be at odds with the concept of facilitating as much independence as possible. Retraining in this setting is important.

Whether a young person with cerebral palsy lives at home with her parents, or by herself, or with another person, she may well need, from time to time, periods of 'short-term' or 'respite' care – to relieve carers or to give those living independently a break. In Britain at present there is a shortage of such care. In childhood these periods of respite care are often spent in another family, but for the young adult, this provision may seem inappropriate.

For young people with cerebral palsy wishing to live independently, one of the problems can be finding enough people (and people with whom the young person can get on) to help with care. Throughout childhood, parents and other carers have seen to their needs, and often the young person has been a passive recipient with little control over how and when the help is offered. It can now be difficult for the young adult to teach new carers and to accept different ways of doing things.

Financial independence is obviously linked with the occupational opportunities of the young person. A great many young people with cerebral palsy in Britain are dependent on state benefits. These generally do not give enough financial freedom for the young person to employ their own carers and decide themselves what help they need. There are a few examples where this does happen, and this must greatly enhance the person's autonomy.

One of the major needs that has been highlighted in many studies is how important mobility is to the quality of life. In terms of independence, it is crucial, and lack of independent mobility is a major factor in the social isolation that affects many young people with disabilities.

6.3 Changing family patterns and establishing adult personal relationships

Social isolation is one of the major findings in different studies of young people with disabilities. Anderson *et al.* (1982) stressed social isolation as their most significant finding and this is certainly borne out in our own experience in Sheffield. Segregation in special schools followed by either placement in special day centres or special units at colleges isolates young people with disabilities from their peer group. Poor mobility and lack of access to leisure pursuits increases the isolation. Friendships tend to grow up within the 'disabled sub-culture'.

Young people with disability often have to rely heavily on parents for transport to social activities, and also, if control of certain aspects of personal hygiene has not been mastered, parents may have to stay around.

Whilst anyone can help a handicapped youngster to wash or dress, only those with a knowledge of practice in appliance fitting can undertake the task of changing the bag. Outside the family it is, of course, rare for anyone to have this knowledge, except for a few professionals. Unless independence is achieved, therefore, the teenager and his parents (often the mother alone) are tied together in a very restrictive way. (Anderson *et al.*, 1982)

Lack of mobility, few friends and dependency on parents, make it hard for the young person to establish an adult role within the family. Often parents may still be in control of the young person's finances, and research has shown that many young people with disabilities do not manage their benefits: 'evidence from a recent survey of severely disabled young people showed that very few managed their own cash benefits and in almost 90% of cases, parents decided how the money would be spent (Hirst, 1985).

Parents have to be helped by professionals to 'let go' of their children with disabilities, and to allow them to take risks. This not only helps the young person but also the parents themselves. If a young person with disabilities still needs help from his parents, this is disabling and restrictive on the parents. By the time their children are reaching adulthood their own elderly parents may be making demands on their time as well, and causing conflict of interest.

Young people with disability who have been to special schools and other segregated settings are at a disadvantage when establishing friendships and contacts in the able-bodied world. They have often not learned the social skills and techniques that are accepted, and peculiar mannerisms and childish behaviour that may have been tolerated in the segregated settings can no longer be so.

There have been a number of experimental studies of interpersonal relations between handicapped and non-handicapped persons . . . The studies deal with short interaction between two persons who have never met, using this design. Hirst (1985) found that subjects who interacted with the person appearing handicapped (1) exhibited more anxiety, (2) distorted their opinions in ways they felt would be more acceptable to the handicapped person, (3) were less spontaneous, (4) showed less variability in their opinions they offered and (5) terminated the meeting sooner. (Richardson, 1972)

Many of the problems already mentioned in this chapter come together and are highlighted in the area of sexuality and disability. The forming of sexual relationships is a major factor in achieving adulthood. There is a preoccupation in modern society with the fit, beautiful body, and this is often linked with sexual desirability. It is difficult to have a positive sexual body image with a disability. Because of the congenital nature of cerebral palsy, the young person will have shared his or her body with doctors and other therapists as well. The body is almost felt to be medical property. Coupled with this, mention is often made of the insensitive handling of examinations in adolescent clinics, e.g. 14/15-year-old girls being examined with groups of medical students in attendance. 'At the age of 14 I had a male physiotherapist and – let me tell you – this is very physically arousing for a healthy 14 year old girl to have a 25 year old male physio. I was a wreck when I left physical therapy – not from pain but from physical anguish, to put it frankly' (Richardson, 1972).

Young people with disabilities often have few opportunities for sexual encounters because of their isolation and dependency on parents. Consequently when there are possibilities, the young people may feel very pressurized.

Most young people receive information on sexual matters at school, backed up by parental input and support. For young people with severe physical disabilities, however, the help/information needed may have to be on a very personal technical level, because of the problems caused by the impairment, e.g. problem of incontinence.

Help in these areas may be beyond the knowledge of parents and teachers and skilled informed help will need to be sought elsewhere. Much written information tends to skate round the subject and talk about 'alternative loving relationships'. Many parents of children with physical disabilities (as do parents of the able-bodied) find it hard to acknowledge their children's sexual needs, but unlike their able-bodied peers, those with disability lack the physical independence to separate from their parents. Young people with disabilities rely heavily on their parents and may accept, consciously or unconsciously, the denial of their sexuality, e.g. age-inappropriate clothes and hair styles. Even if later on independence is achieved, the psychological effect of this denial can lead to many problems. It seems sad that many young people with disabilities feel sexual activity is 'more trouble than it's worth'.

At present, many young people with disabilities socialize in the main within the 'disabled sub-culture' – hence help is often needed to have sexual intercourse, help with undressing and comfortable positioning. This requires a great deal of emotional ability on behalf of the helpers and helped alike, and can cause conflicts in 'institutionalized' settings, e.g. between parents of the young people and their professional carers. Spontaneity, often an important element in sexual activity, is virtually impossible in some cases. Also for those who are severely disabled, sexual activity may be very tiring. This caring relationship may not be the norm in young adult relationships. Many young couples with disabilities may dismiss the idea of having a family because of their inability to rear children independently. If both partners are disabled there is a guilt feeling of having to ask for outside help; where the female partner has disabilities she may feel that the able-bodied partner will have to bear an inordinate amount of care of the child, as well as the continued care of the mother.

If it is accepted that people with disabilities have the same rights as the 'able-bodied' then help must be given in such a way as to reduce these feelings. Care must also be readily available and delivered in a flexible way. Initial genetic counselling and information about the effect of pregnancy and childbirth on a woman with disabilities must also be available.

6.4   Establishing a role and participating in the community

Where young people with disabilities have not been able to become independent, it is often hard for them to establish an adult role in the community. Because of the segregation of services, the general public have little personal knowledge of and contact with people with disabilities: 'Isolation is the prime breeding ground of myths and stereotypes' (McConkey and McCormack, 1983).

The contact that there is is often distorted – and portrays a charitable image – 'The commitment of disability organisations to community education is often blunted by other demands. Public support for their fund-raising activities is most easily enlisted by emphasising the inadequacies of their handicapped clients'. This picture maintains the person with disabilities as being always a recipient of services and not contributing to the community. There is also an enormous gulf in knowledge between the professional and the general public, which has led to major difficulties when talking about community care. As well as the increased contact that must be brought about by more integrated settings, there is a need for a planned effective programme, not only of education of the public about disability in general and about particular needs of people with disabilities, but also to bring groups together to meet and discuss problems facing both the able-bodied and disabled and hence emphasizing the similarities and not just the differences.

A great many self-help and pressure groups of people with disabilities have been established and are playing a much greater part in planning services – not just those for people with disabilities but those services that are used by all – seeking to ensure that the needs of people with disabilities are taken into account.

Professionals concerned with young adults with cerebral palsy and other disabilities must push hard to teach the young people how to become their own advocates, and must also advocate on their behalf if necessary. There is no point in pouring therapeutic services into children with cerebral palsy if it is to lead to an environmentally impoverished and isolated adulthood. The aim of all parents and professionals involved with young people with disabilities has to be to help them to take their place in the adult world with as much dignity and independence as is possible.

It is to be hoped that in the future no young person with a disability will feel like making comments such as the following: 'I thought you would wait until I am dead before you buried me' (Kent *et al.*, 1984).

PART THREE
Assessment and Therapy

Introduction

This final section aims to highlight the broad issues involved in the assessment and facilitation procedures for the child and young person with cerebral palsy. Some aspects of assessment and treatment are common to all.

1. Effective treatment must be preceded by thorough relevant and expert assessment of the child's status, potential, rate of learning and needs.
2. Parents must be involved at all stages of information gathering and decision making if they are to feel empowered to work with and help their child.
3. The rationale behind assessment and therapy will change over time. In the neonate and young child the emphasis will be on development and the attainment of maximum potential. In the older child and young person the more important issues to emerge will be those of enablement; of making the most of current skills; of equipment and technology to maintain function.

7   Sensory assessment: hearing and vision

7.1   Hearing impairment in children with cerebral palsy

It is imperative to make a full assessment of the child's hearing ability for several reasons. The cerebral insults which are sufficient to produce permanent impairment within the motor system may simultaneously damage the cochlea, and possibly the brainstem nuclei (Hall, 1964; Pape and Wigglesworth, 1979). As a result, severe sensori-neural deafness is a common additional handicap in four limb involvement cerebral palsy and particularly in athetoid or dyskinetic cerebral palsy (Newton, 1985). Secondly, a hearing impairment in a child with a physical disability who may also have an attention deficit and/or learning difficulties, is likely to have a more profound effect on the child's learning of speech and language than would be the case in the absence of physical disability.

7.1.1   METHODS

The detection of hearing impairment in infants is normally attempted when it is possible to carry out a simple behavioural test (localization of sound). This test is usually performed at about 8 months of age. This test, currently employed in population screening, requires considerable care and only works well when a high and sustained level of training is provided for the tester (McCormick, 1983). Other reports, however (Newton, 1985), indicate that the behavioural test may be inadequate, detecting only 55% of cases of hearing impairment in screened populations. The advantage of a good reproducible distraction test in a child is that: (a) information about threshold and frequency range are obtained and (b) the child displays an appropriate response to sound (i.e. by turning to the stimulus). Hence all children with cerebral palsy who are over 4 months old are examined by distraction testing in the first instance, followed by tympanometry. Children with unsatisfactory or doubtful results are further investigated by brain stem electric response testing (BSER).

Table 7.1   Incidence of visual defects in cerebral palsy

	Marguelec 1966 (%)	*Henderson 1961 (%)*
Squint	22	35
Gaze palsy	—	1.8
Nystagmus	8	13
Cataract	—	1.2
Optic atrophy	9	9.9

(a)   BSER testing

In this test the changes in the EEG signal in response to auditory stimuli are recorded. The method is well described by Stevens *et al.* (1987). Four standard silver/silver chloride electrodes are placed on the mastoid process, the vertex and the forehead (ground). Ipsilateral recordings are made between each mastoid electrode and the vertex electrode. The EEG signal is amplified and averaged and stored on a microcomputer, which also controls the auditory stimulator. The stimuli are 100 µs unipolar compression clicks delivered into an ear-phone as used in electrocochleography. Two thousand sweeps at each stimulus level are used. By this means it is possible to establish the threshold of EEG response to auditory stimuli across a broad frequency range. Children who do not display normal responses bilaterally are referred for further audiological investigation and, if necessary, the fitting of hearing aids.

7.2   Visual impairment in children with cerebral palsy

Children with cerebral palsy are at high risk of an associated visual disorder. At the Ryegate Children's Centre 48% of children with cerebral palsy were found to have a visual defect; this compares to a figure of approximately 4–5% for the child population generally (Shentall and Hosking, 1986). In a study of 382 cases of cerebral palsy, Marguelec found 19% of the children to be partially or completely blind, 27% had refractive errors, 22% had various forms of squint, 8% of the children had nystagmus and 9% optic atrophy (Marguelec, 1966). Henderson's classic treatise on cerebral palsy contains considerable detail of ophthalmic disorders (Henderson, 1961). Some data from these studies are compared in Table 7.1. It is clear that full visual assessment is mandatory for children with cerebral palsy.

7.2.1   VISUAL ASSESSMENT

There are numerous problems that may render a visual assessment more difficult in the child with cerebral palsy:

1. Poor seating or play position making cooperation difficult.
2. Difficulty in communication (child).
3. Cognitive impairment. The child may not use vision because of perceptual and intellectual difficulties even though vision itself may be normal.

In children with severe learning difficulties behavioural problems may also impair the response to testing.

7.2.2   AIDS TO ASSESSMENT

A good idea of a child's visual function can be obtained by simple observation during free play or therapy. A single presentation of a toy prevents confusion, but a variety of toys that can be used in assessment is necessary. Conventional test materials can be presented along with play material, e.g. graded rolling balls, Sheridan Gardner letter matching, Kay picture naming test, small toy matching, ability to see small sweets, etc. In the more mature child the more formal presentation of test materials is possible.

7.2.3   EVOKED RESPONSE TESTING

In children in whom informal and formal conventional assessment is very difficult or impossible, further information about the integrity of the visual system can be obtained by evoked response testing (Stephenson and King, 1989). The other main application of these tests is in the diagnostic assessment of the primary neurological disease. In this situation evoked potential recording can be diagnostic of certain conditions. The tests depend upon the recording of electrical signals from surface electrodes. These potentials can be recorded from the retina (electroretinogram – ERG) or from the visual cortex (visual evoked potentials – VEP).

The ERG is recorded using a surface electrode at the nasion or a gold foil electrode placed on the lower eyelid. The ERG can be of considerable interest in situations where an evaluation of retinal function is required. For example, diminution or absence of the ERG will be found in the preclinical stages of disorders of the superficial layers of the retina, particularly retinitis pigmentosa.

The VEP response is similar in some respects to the auditory brain response – the signal is detected by placing an electrode over the visual cortex and computer averaging the EEG signal produced in response to a repetitive light signal (flash). A VEP may also be obtained by stimulating with a pattern (e.g. a chequerboard). In the early stages of retinitis pigmentosa, while the ERG may be absent, the VEP will initially at least be normal. As the disorder progresses the VEP will become abnormal. Abnormality of the VEP will occur in any disorder affecting the visual system from the ganglion cell of the retina to the visual cortex and it should be remembered that in the child with cerebral palsy there may be more than one lesion (e.g. optic atrophy and occipital periventricular leucomalacia). These visual studies should always be regarded as adjuncts to the clinical assessment of the child and not absolute tests of visual function – they provide important diagnostic information in certain circumstances, only very rarely can they answer the question 'Can my child see?'

8 *Epilepsy and cerebral palsy*

8.1 Incidence and classification

Cerebral palsy has been described in earlier chapters as a group of clinical syndromes caused by damage to the immature brain. The associated problems of learning difficulties and communication disorders have also been described in some detail. A further manifestation of cerebral injury is epilepsy.

Epilepsy may co-exist with cerebral palsy. Epilepsy may be defined as a condition in which there are recurrent, paroxysmal attacks of unconsciousness or altered consciousness, often in association with tonic or clonic muscle contraction and/or altered behaviour. In practice, many synonyms are used in discussions about epilepsy, such as 'fits', 'seizures', 'convulsions' and 'epileptic attacks'.

Epilepsy is a common and often disabling additional problem in children with cerebral palsy. The incidence of epilepsy in populations of children with cerebral palsy is variable (Ingram, 1964; Hagberg *et al.*, 1975). The incidence observed in the study of Sheffield children (1980–6) referred to in Part One is compared in Table 8.1 with the composite figures quoted by Aicardi (1990) from a variety of studies. Corbett and Pond (1985) report an overall incidence of 36% of children with cerebral palsy having recurrent seizures and comment that the children with the highest incidence of seizures are those in whom associated mental handicap was most severe. Over a ten-year follow-up period epilepsy was the commonest cause of death in the children with cerebral palsy and severe learning difficulties. These incidence figures compare with population figures for non cerebral palsied children where the figure is in the order 0.5–0.7% (Aicardi, 1980).

Two further points should be noted. Firstly the children with cerebral palsy who have seizures are at much higher risk of learning difficulties. This point is well made in the case of hemiplegia, where severe learning difficulties were more frequently observed in the children with hemiplegia and epilepsy (Sussova *et al.*, 1990). Also, in hemiplegic epilepsy there may be a slow decline of intelligence, often with increasing behavioural problems which can be very resistant to

Table 8.1 Incidence of epilepsy in cerebral palsy

Clinical type of CP	Frequency of epilepsy	
	Sheffield (%)	Various studies* (%)
Spastic hemiplegia	25	34–60
Spastic diplegia	7	16–27
Spastic quadriplegia	43	50–90
Ataxic	0	—
Dyskinetic	—	23–26

* Aicardi (1990).

therapy (Lindsay *et al.*, 1987). In children with four limb involvement cerebral palsy due to severe bilateral hemisphere damage or malformation with frequent seizures (perhaps many seizures per day) the effect of the seizures on intelligence can be very difficult to assess but is likely to be significant. Such children frequently require vigorous drug therapy and often do not respond well to single drug management so that the medication may contribute to the learning problems (Foley, 1990).

The second point is that in some cases of cerebral palsy the motor handicap may be relatively mild but the epilepsy severely disabling, causing intellectual, behavioural and social handicaps far in excess of the movement disorder.

Epileptic seizures are classified according to the clinical attack and most authorities attempt to follow the international classification of epilepsy (Gastaut, 1981). In practice such precise classification is often very difficult, especially in the description of various forms of partial seizures (Bax, 1990).

International Classification of Epilepsy

1. Partial seizures
   (a) simple partial seizures
       (i) with motor signs
       (ii) with somato-sensory or special sensory hallucinations
       (iii) with autonomic symptoms and signs
       (iv) with psychic symptoms
   (b) complex partial seizures
       (i) simple partial onset then impaired consciousness

      (ii) with impaired consciousness at onset

   (c) partial seizures evolving to secondary generalized seizures

      (i) simple partial seizures evolving to generalized

      (ii) complex partial to generalized

      (iii) simple partial to complex partial to generalized.

2. Generalized seizures

   (a) (i) absence seizures

       (ii) atypical absence

   (b) myoclonic seizures

   (c) clonic seizures

   (d) tonic seizures

   (e) tonic-clonic seizures

   (f) atonic seizures.

3. Unclassifiable seizures.

In a child with cerebral palsy and epilepsy the epileptic attacks may fall within any of the above types, that is there is no single seizure type typical of cerebral injury. However it is unusual to encounter primary generalized seizures in children with cerebral palsy, most often the seizure type is of the complex partial variety or partial evolving to secondary generalized.

During a partial seizure, at least at the outset, only part of the brain is involved in the abnormal electrical discharge. Symptomatology is dependent upon the site of origin of the discharge – in the case of the motor cortex the abnormal discharge may provoke abnormal muscle contraction (this is in fact very uncommon) – if the abnormal discharge arises in the temporal lobe then there may be severe disruption of perception and emotion, which the child may describe vividly, or alternatively may provoke bizarre behavioural displays. These episodes are often referred to as temporal lobe attacks or temporal lobe epilepsy (TLE).

In a generalized seizure the abnormal electrical activity is present throughout the brain and thus many more areas of brain activity are overwhelmed by the episode, and so consciousness is always affected. The child may not be aware of any abnormality, however – in childhood absence epilepsy (Petit Mal) the child immediately recovers and may resume previous activities without any apparent interruption in processing. In more dramatic generalized seizures the child will be aware that something has happened but will be unable to describe the episode with accuracy. In a number of cases in which partial seizures progress to become secondary generalized seizures, the child will be able to describe the initial but not the later aspects of the attack.

8.2 Management

The development of epileptic seizures in a child with cerebral palsy is always a profoundly disturbing occurrence. As professionals, we are usually not surprised to hear the description of the child's first seizure, but the event carries the same impact with the child's family as it would with the non-handicapped child. The two main tasks at this point are as follows.

1. Is it certain that the attack(s) are epileptic?
2. What do the parents know about epilepsy and what do they need to know?

The first question can be extremely difficult, especially in those cases where the parents have not yet witnessed an attack and are relying on accounts from another. In these circumstances it is essential that the physician obtain a first hand account of the episode before making further management decisions. Secondly, the recording of the electro-encephalogram (EEG) may give important diagnostic information. Most often, however, the interictal EEG in children with cerebral palsy will not resolve this question when clinical information is insufficient to reach a decision.

In those cases where the diagnosis of epilepsy is clear, the second task of informing the parents and the child must now commence. In particular the parents will have many questions concerning all aspects of epileptic seizures; their origins, complications, treatment and outcome. Considerable time will need to be taken in discussion of these issues, but it is also extremely helpful to have written information available which can be absorbed at leisure and later discussed with the physician (e.g. *The Epilepsy Reference Book*, Jeavons and Aspinall, 1985).

Most parents will wish for some attempt to be made to prevent further episodes occurring. Three areas will need some consideration in children with epilepsy and cerebral palsy:

1. Avoidance of environmental precipitant, if any.
2. Drug treatment (including use of ketogenic diet).
3. Surgical treatment.

It is always necessary to consider any environmental influence, although this will rarely be relevant. For the most part treatment of the epilepsy means anticonvulsant medication. Most paediatricians in the UK would hesitate to treat with anticonvulsant drugs a child after the first seizure, unless the seizure was prolonged, particularly unpleasant, or followed by post-ictal paralysis. In most cases two or more seizures require the administration of an anticonvulsant drug, especially if the seizures occur after a relatively short interval. Many authorities in the field of epilepsy and its treatment take the view that seizures should be suppressed by treatment as soon as possible. This recommendation is founded on the observation that the frequency of untreated seizures tends to increase, suggesting a decrease in the threshold for further seizures (Reynolds, 1987). An alternative view is occasionally valid in those children who have infrequent minor seizures and who also have severe learning difficulties. In this situation the adverse effects of anticonvulsant medication on learning can be very difficult to discern in the clinical setting, and a decision to 'wait and see' may be appropriate.

The selection of a particular anticonvulsant drug for the child will depend on several factors, most important of which are: likely efficacy in the seizure type, acceptability in terms of dosing and formulation (both to child and family), the need for anticonvulsant drug blood level monitoring and possible side effects. It is not possible in this short review to deal with the various options in drug selection, except to say that the primary aim is to achieve satisfactory seizure control using a single agent in the lowest dose. Incremental increases are advised until control is achieved, or it can be concluded that the agent is ineffective, or the side effects are unacceptable. In generalized epilepsy sodium valproate seems to be the most effective, particularly in juvenile myoclonic epilepsy. In the treatment of the various partial seizures no particular drug has been shown to be superior. However in the UK most paediatricians select either sodium valproate or carbamazepine. Phenytoin can be very effective in this situation, but its use requires close monitoring of blood levels to ensure efficacy and avoid toxicity. Phenobarbitone, ethosuximide and the benzodiazepines may be used but are usually regarded as second line agents and tend to have an increased incidence of side effects. Vigabatrin, a newly introduced drug acting on the GABA system, seems to show particular effectiveness in complex partial seizures as an add-on medication where single drug treatment has been ineffective.

In children who continue to have frequent and disabling seizures in spite of adequate medication, consideration can be given to the use of a ketogenic diet. This form of treatment followed the observation of remission of seizures in patients who were ketotic (Wilder, 1921). Much has been written since on this interesting subject (Huttenlocher, 1976; Schwartz *et al.*, 1989) and various methods described for inducing ketosis. Commonly the diet comprises a high fat intake combined with a reduction in carbohydrate intake. In some children with refractory seizures the diet can be very effective in reducing seizure frequency, but it can also be difficult to maintain patient compliance and satis-factory growth (Schwartz *et al.*, 1989).

Finally in a very small group of children with disabling epilepsy, most often that seen in association with hemiplegia, consideration should be given to epilepsy surgery for those refractory to drug treat-ment. The number of children who are selected for surgery remains small in the UK at the time of writing. However, the results are thus far encouraging in terms of seizure frequency and post surgical morbidity (Lindsay *et al.*, 1987).

9 *Mobility*

Movement is an essential basic ability necessary to make the best use of all other faculties, to react to surroundings, to explore and to learn. Maria Montessori (1910) saw movement as an expression of personality:

> Thought and action are two parts of the same occurrence. A child uses his movements to extend his understanding. Behaviour is compounded of purposeful movement to a social end.

While normal children, through curiosity, will seek their own sensory stimulation, many children with cerebral palsy will need help to see, feel, smell and to develop their repertoire of experiences. It may be that movement is not pleasurable to the child with cerebral palsy. It may cause pain or be unfamiliar and distressing. Normal babies learn by repetition of movements which they find pleasurable, and absence of pleasure can facilitate a vicious circle of malachievement (Fig. 9.1).

9.1 Assessment of mobility

The nature and emphasis of assessment will vary according to the child's age and ability but essentially the assessment process will gather the following information.

1. Identification of the needs of the child and his family.
2. Formulation of a profile of the child's strengths, abilities and disabilities.
3. Identification of how the child functions within his environment, e.g. home, school, community.
4. Formulation and definition of objectives in relation to the child and the family's needs.

Although assessment changes in its emphasis according to age and ability, it should retain core elements common to all stages of development, and these will be discussed firstly.

Information vital to the assessment can be gathered by the physiotherapist during case history taking, but may also be available from

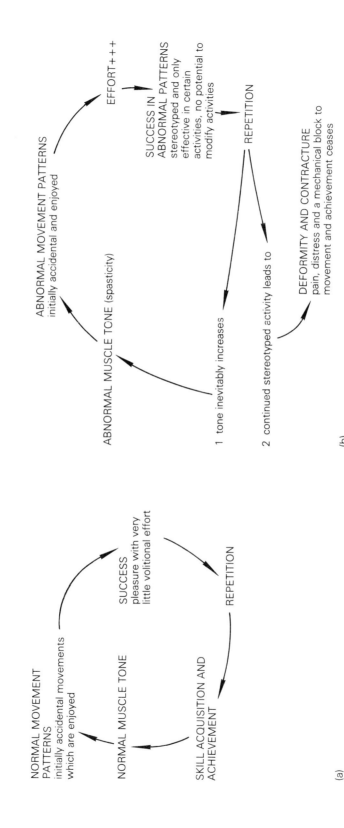

Fig. 9.1 (a) The continuous cycle of achievement and (b) the vicious cycle of malachievement.

the assessments of other members of the multidisciplinary team. Such information will include medical history, current drug therapy, social circumstances, the family's attitude to the child's disability, and their interpretation of the main problems and needs. In addition, the physiotherapist will need other developmental information about hearing, vision, sensory loss or hypersensitivity, communication, feeding and cognitive development.

9.1.1 THE OBJECTIVE EXAMINATION

This involves the collection of physical data through observation and palpation of the child. It forms the bulk of the assessment and aims to determine the degree of dysfunction. The objective examination can be sub-categorized into the following.

(a) Observation

(i) Parent–child interaction Much can be learnt purely by observing how the parent and child interact and interrelate, which may often be done during the history taking so that parent and child are unaware of the assessment. It is useful to observe a small child on the parent's lap and it is important to note factors such as:

1. anxiety: is the child nervous, irritable, upset by the situation, and is the parent showing signs of anxiety?
2. communication: how does the child communicate with his parents, do they share eye contact and smiles, is there conversation or vocalization, does the child use movement to communicate, e.g. extensor thrust or body language?
3. handling skills: it is important to watch parent handling – are the parents sensitive to the child's movements, do they adapt and change handling in accordance with the child's position, do they adapt their positioning of the child automatically to enable him to function better, e.g. repositioning a child with extensor thrust in an upright sitting position to enable him to play with a toy?
4. observation of the child being undressed: how does the child respond to movement, is he stiff, floppy, able/unable to aid activity, or independent, does he find movement painful or distressing? It is also very useful to watch the parents' approach to moving the child. Does the parent provide instruction with the activity, does he/she handle and move the child sensitively, and does the parent adapt the handling according to physical changes and cues from the child, e.g. it may be best to handle a stiff spastic child slowly and precisely, so as not to increase muscle tone, although some parents

may pull at the child's limbs indiscriminately despite the child's response? It is also common to observe overprotection of the child during undressing, the parent performing more of the task for the child than is necessary, not allowing him to function at full potential.

(ii) Observation of the child This is best carried out when the child is undressed, or in as little clothing as possible. It is best if the child is on the floor with plenty of space, although there should be furniture close at hand for the child to use if necessary. There should be a selection of age-appropriate toys within reach.

Initially the child is observed on the floor without intervention.

1. Movement: the following need to be explored. Does the child stay where he is placed, unable to move from the initial position? Is the child able to move but unable to change position? Does the child exhibit normal or abnormal patterns of movement? It is necessary to describe what the child is able to do and how, particularly if the movement is abnormal. Is the child able to change position from that in which he is initially placed? For instance, can the child roll from supine to prone? If so, how does he perform the activity? Does he use abnormal muscle tone and reflex activity to perform the skill? How does the ability to move compare with developmental norms for the child? If the child shows a marked asymmetry, it is necessary to describe the nature of this, for instance, asymmetrical tonic neck reflex (ATNR), spasticity increased one side more than the other. Has the child retained pathological reflex activity, e.g. ATNR, tonic labyrinthine reflex, startle, reflex etc.? Again, if so, it is useful to describe how this interferes with movement. Does the child demonstrate equilibrium and balance reactions?
2. Play: can the child move to, and does he choose to move to, toys (sensory deficits may be a factor here)? It should be noted what sort of toy the child chooses to play with, and his manipulation of them should be observed and described. Does the child choose a more or less sophisticated toy than would be normal for his age? Does the effort or excitement of play affect the child's overall muscle tone?
3. Tone: by the end of the observational assessment, the therapist will have a good idea of how the child's muscle tone will feel on palpation. As normal muscle tone is the basis of normal movement, it is important to have an accurate assessment of the basic postural tone and this can be carried out during the observational assessment as described, and also through observation with intervention.

(b) Observation with intervention

In this part of the assessment the physiotherapist handles and moves the child in order to observe him in differing positions – supine, prone, side lying, sitting and standing. In the more capable child, walking, running, jumping and more sophisticated motor activities are observed and facilitated.

Again it should be noted how the child performs activities. Where motor activities are abnormal the therapist will try to facilitate a normal approach.

The physiotherapist will experiment with ways to facilitate position changes and inhibit abnormal movements interfering with motor functioning. This will affect muscle tone and successful handling methods producing a positive response should be noted.

At this point assessment is very closely linked with treatment, and the two are interdependent. Attempts at treatment by positioning the child in different ways must be assessed for effectiveness and that information used to develop new treatment plans.

(c) Contracture and deformity

Because contracture and deformity are often present with cerebral palsy, particularly in older children, assessment of the young child should take note of 'danger' areas following examination of range of movement and movement patterns, e.g. tight adductors, tight hamstrings, etc. These problems should then be addressed.

In the older child where contracture is already established, these must be noted with accuracy to enable comparison to be made at later assessments, and to ensure that impossible goals are not set for the child in treatment planning.

(d) The use of developmental milestones in assessment

It is important to have a knowledge of 'vertical' developmental milestones when assessing the child with cerebral palsy. However, it is also important to realize that developmental milestones may not always be useful when dealing with a child who may never achieve more than, for example, minimal head control.

9.1.2. INTERPRETATION OF THE FINDINGS

The objective of the initial examination is to arrive at an assessment of the child's dysfunction, from which therapy pertinent to that child's needs can be formulated.

As the child matures and reaches adulthood, the emphasis of care shifts. For those young adults with little or no intellectual impairment,

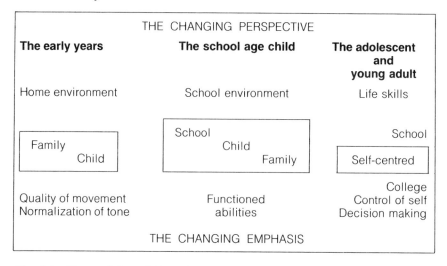

Fig. 9.2   The evolving philosophies of care.

the approach becomes more self-orientated. By this age most will have chosen which method of mobility they feel suits them best. They will have decided about college or work placements, and again the therapist will become involved in helping to adapt the environment and helping them to adapt, so as to enable optimum functioning. The fundamental aspects of quality of normal movements are still observed, however. At this stage the physiotherapist may use an abnormal movement, which may have persisted despite all efforts, in order to produce function.

For the young adult with more severe intellectual impairment, care may tend to shift back to the parents. As the young person comes to school leaving age, some may enter college or adult training centre, but facilities are restricted. The physiotherapist will continue to be involved in a supportive and functional way, helping the young adult to adapt and function optimally within his environment.

Figure 9.2 demonstrates the changing perspective of assessment and treatment of the child and later young adult with cerebral palsy over the years.

9.2   Treatment

In the early stages physiotherapy must be aimed at interrupting the vicious circle of malachievement caused by abnormal muscle tone. By helping to normalize tone, it may be possible to ameliorate the consequences of this circle.

It is clear that amelioration of these movement patterns cannot be achieved in one treatment session once a week, where the child is removed from his normal surroundings to be handled 'correctly' by a physiotherapist for short periods in a brief therapeutic situation. Physiotherapy should rather aim to orientate the child's family to a way of handling, a way of carrying out everyday tasks, which becomes the 'norm'.

The parents should be exposed to correct handling of their child. The physiotherapist can demonstrate how correct handling can fit into normal routine and can illustrate those positions and movements which should be encouraged and those which are contraindicated. The parents should become expert in handling their child, the therapist's role being that of a teacher or adviser, continually adapting the handling and management as appropriate and supporting and encouraging the parents.

Eventually as the child matures and goes to school, teachers and other carers become involved, and the same advice and encouragement should continue to ensure a consistent approach. Ultimately, the goal is for the person with cerebral palsy to be responsible for his own movement patterns, to participate in normal life skills and activities in as free and normal a way as possible.

9.3 Neurodevelopmental treatment of the child with cerebral palsy

In the face of a disorder which by definition is a permanent motor deficit, many approaches to therapy have been developed. All of these therapies have at times attracted considerable interest and almost evangelical supporters, and on one occasion equally evangelical opponents. Only relatively recently have attempts been made to evaluate the merits of different approaches. The methodological difficulties encountered in such studies mean that it may be some time before sound data are acquired which show clearly the most useful approaches.

No single approach will suit all children with whatever form of cerebral palsy. It is our firm view that the proposed management of the child should be based on a full assessment of the whole child and family. We favour an 'eclectic' style of therapy which draws upon a variety of techniques and methods rather than the devout pursuit of a single technique. This practice seems eminently sensible from a professional point of view. There are sometimes problems, however, as the approach is perhaps less easily seen as a 'technique'. On occasions a single minded application of a 'method' may seem more attractive to parents, perhaps because a method appears like a treatment and as such carries the aura of greater effectiveness (cure). This is an area where much is said and argued over but where there is little hard data. The few attempts at controlled studies that have so far been undertaken have shown mixed results (e.g. Herndon *et al.*, 1987; Palmer *et al.*, 1988; Tirosh and Rabino, 1989). There follows a brief account of the most interesting approaches currently available (the reader should consult the source material for more detailed descriptions of the different techniques).

9.3.1   THE NEURODEVELOPMENTAL APPROACH

The ideas and work of Bertha Bobath have had the most profound effect on the training and practice of physiotherapists in the United Kingdom and in certain parts of the USA. Much of the method employed by therapists at the Rycgate Children's Centre owes its development to the principles she has laid down.

In the normal infant, muscle tone varies with posture and the infant's movements comprise, to a large extent, the primary 'reflex' responses. As cortical control of movement develops, these responses are progressively integrated into the child's developing volitional schema of movement; the movements the child displays become less predictable and reflexive but the primary responses are not discarded, rather incorporated into more complex movement patterns. In the normal child this cortical influence inhibits all but the required movement, but in the child with cerebral palsy this influence is lessened, which leads to the persistence and dominance of the primary responses. This in turn leads to the disorder of posture and movement (Fig. 9.3).

The aims of treatment using the Bobath approaches are as follows (Bobath, 1963).

1. To change the child's abnormal postural patterns in order to give him a more normal postural background for his movements.
2. To reduce hypertonus, i.e. spasticity or intermittent spasms, so that movement becomes effortless and pleasurable, and to increase muscle tone in flaccid, athetoid and ataxic patients so that postures against gravity can be maintained, fixation given to movement and every range of movement controlled by balanced contraction and relaxation of agonists and antagonists.
3. To develop the most important fundamental movement patterns, such as head control, turning over, sitting up, kneeling, standing and balance reactions in all positions and activities.

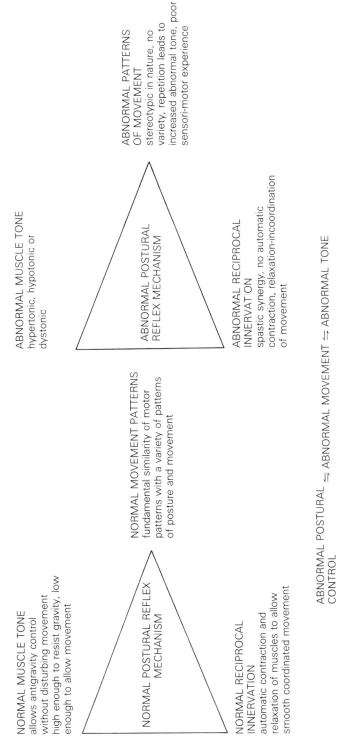

NORMAL MUSCLE TONE
allows antigravity control
without disturbing movement
high enough to resist gravity, low
enough to allow movement

NORMAL MOVEMENT PATTERNS
fundamental similarity of motor
patterns with a variety of patterns
of posture and movement

ABNORMAL MUSCLE TONE
hypertonic, hypotonic or
dystonic

ABNORMAL PATTERNS
OF MOVEMENT
stereotypic in nature, no
variety, repetition leads to
increased abnormal tone, poor
sensori-motor experience

NORMAL POSTURAL REFLEX
MECHANISM

ABNORMAL POSTURAL
REFLEX MECHANISM

NORMAL RECIPROCAL
INNERVATION
automatic contraction and
relaxation of muscles to allow
smooth coordinated movement

ABNORMAL RECIPROCAL
INNERVATION
spastic synergy, no automatic
contraction, relaxation-incoordination
of movement

ABNORMAL POSTURAL ⇆ ABNORMAL MOVEMENT ⇆ ABNORMAL TONE
CONTROL

Fig. 9.3 The relationship between muscle tone, movement and posture.

4. To teach skilled motor patterns for everyday life and self-help. Bobath's method emphasized the importance of improving coordination of posture and movement and maintaining a more normal muscle tone. She believed that a more normal postural reflex mechanism is a prerequisite for normal movement. A normal background of muscle tone for movement should be sufficiently high to make weight-bearing against gravity possible and to give fixation to movement, but it must not be so high as to interfere with movement. Changes of posture are necessary accompaniments to movement and take place before movement begins. Every movement therefore requires a 'postural set' to make it possible and more easy to perform, and in children with cerebral palsy their 'postural sets' make many movements impossible. The child cannot initiate movement by altering his posture and cannot adapt his posture during a movement. Much work should therefore be aimed at normalizing muscle tone by inhibiting postural reflex activity.

'Before he can be expected to do a certain movement, we should make sure that his muscle tone is sufficiently normal to allow the movement to be performed in at least a fairly normal way. The child is helped and guided . . . rather than allowed to struggle by himself.' It is this point that has given rise to some important criticism of the approach – therapists feeling that the intensive 'hands on' aspect should be modified to allow greater choice and determination by the child. Nancie Finnie has produced an excellent description of the practical application of the neurodevelopmental approach to the daily management of the child (Finnie, 1974).

9.3.2   TEMPLE FAY AND THE INSTITUTE FOR THE ADVANCEMENT OF HUMAN POTENTIAL

Dr Temple Fay (1946) developed an approach to the management of the effects of cerebral injury from the standpoint of the neurophysiologist. His propositions for management reflected a deep interest in the evolutionary aspects of locomotor development, hence:

The nervous system represents a series of evolutionary levels of functional development. When higher centres are out of control, the simple patterns of movement seen in early infancy must be learned well before attempting the more complex patterns of crawling and walking. We have placed much emphasis on the . . . 'fish crawl' because it represents the movements most common to the amphibians. The patient is placed on the abdomen and the arm and the leg of the same side (homolateral pattern) are drawn up together, flexed and made ready to extend in a sweeping movement out to the side (alligator crawl), meanwhile, the opposite arm and leg are extended (having finished their act). Alternating extension and flexion of the extremities are begun in a swimming–crawling fashion. The head should take on an alternating movement face–chin to the side being extended, and occiput to the side about to be flexed.

Doman *et al.*, 1960 took up these ideas, extended and developed them with additional rather dubious techniques including rebreathing into a plastic bag ('to improve cerebral blood flow') and suspending the child upside down (same rationale). Some families have reported good outcomes from this approach but many have been distressed and disturbed by the approach. At the Ryegate Children's Centre we try to dissuade parents from developing an interest in this technique because we feel that the approach is theoretically unsound with its heavy reliance on involuntary movements to 'pattern' the child's volitional movement. We subscribe to the view that whatever approach is advocated there must be a strong emphasis on developing the child's *voluntary* movement. Secondly, the technique is highly invasive to the child and severely disrupts the child's and family's opportunities to enjoy everyday experiences.

9.3.3 CONDUCTIVE EDUCATION

Conductive education is the approach developed by Dr Andras Peto (1903–1967) at the National Motor Therapy Institute in Budapest; it is a system of rehabilitation that has excited much interest in recent years. There is no doubt that the approach is unique and deserves serious examination. Many British children and their families now make the journey to Hungary to undergo assessment and management at the Institute. Following the upsurge of interest in the technique in the early 1980s, a British centre (in Birmingham) was established, run on similar lines and with guidance from the Hungarian institute.

The method has a number of easily identifiable characteristics.

1. There is relatively little special equipment. That which is used is most often apparatus such as the ladderback chair and the slatted plinth. Splinting, fixing and bracing are not in common use, wheelchairs are not employed, and sticks are used only occasionally. The emphasis is on 'orthofunction', which seems to mean the ability to be continent, to walk and to cope with stairs, and to write.
2. Activities are mainly group-based. Groups vary in size and there may be up to 20–25 children in each. A lot of emphasis is placed on the performance of the child in the group, and also the effect of the group on the child. The groups are, as far as possible, matched for age, disability and ability.

3. Conductors are staff trained over a four-year course and are unique to the Institute. It is they who run the groups and make all the decisions about the childrens' activities.
4. Rhythmic intention: music is a curriculum subject in all Hungarian schools, and Peto incorporated music and rhythm in the programmes he developed for rehabilitation. One aspect which is important in this area is the aspect of rhythmic intention – the rhythmic/musical vocalizing of the description of the movement as the movement is performed or attempted.
5. Volition: great emphasis is placed on the child's drive and personal desire to achieve the allotted task. Passive movement or exercise is not a feature of the system.
6. Intensity: children from the age of 3 years or so are resident for academic terms at the Institute, and so are exposed to the rehabilitation technique throughout their whole day.

Considerable claims have been made for the success of the approach (though not noticeably from the staff of the Institute). The Institute has released a number of fascinating statistics relating to the rate of children discharged from the Institute who are orthofunctional. The figure is usually in the order 65–75%. The difficulty in assessing these data has been alluded to in Chapter 1. It is quite probable that there will be differences between the distribution of types of disorder in Hungary and those predominating in the United Kingdom, and so it will not be possible to draw valid comparison with groups in the United Kingdom or the USA. Also the Institute does not take on all children referred; a number of children will be thought unsuitable (15% of referred cases) (Cottam and Sutton, 1986), due to severe learning difficulties, severe epilepsy or blindness. It is pertinent here to refer to the data produced by Crothers and Paine (1959), which gave independent walking rates for 289 children with cerebral palsy tabulated against age at walking. These data show an independent walking rate at age 7 years for hemiplegia of nearly 100%, for extrapyramidal and mixed types of 70%, and for spastic quadriplegics of 67%.

These methods are the major approaches under discussion and in use at the present time in the United Kingdom. It is very likely that we shall see substantial growth in the development and application of conductive education during the coming decade.

9.4   Contracture and deformity in cerebral palsy

The threat of contractures and deformity of joints can be noted very early when spasticity is present. These symptoms are the result of asymmetry within the body or the constant use of spasticity for functional activity. Children most prone to deformity are those with spastic quadriplegia, especially when there is severe asymmetry. However, all types of children with cerebral palsy are subject to risk if spasticity for movement continues. For instance, those at risk include the diplegic child who bunny hops for mobility and who 'W' sits, i.e. with legs to either side, and the hemiplegic child not encouraged to use the affected side for function. Figure 9.4 shows some of the common causes of deformity and contracture.

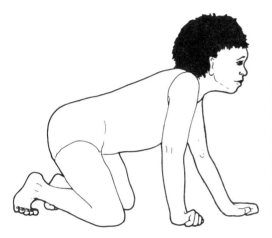

'Bunny hopping'
Spastic diplegic children often bunny hop for mobility. In doing so they use alternating flexor and extensor spasticity and abnormal symmetrical tonic neck reflex to be mobile – this is a typical 'flexion for function' activity common to diplegics. If encouraged and not controlled, it will reduce the potential for the child in standing and walking, causing increased flexion and ultimately contracture of hip and knee flexors. The posture also encourages increased plantar flexion of ankles and TA tightness

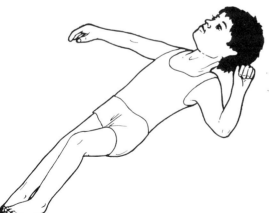

The asymmetrical tonic neck reflex
This is often seen in more severe spastic quadriplegic children in whom the reflex is obligatory. Continued stereotyped posturing means the child may not bring hands together and gain hand–eye coordination, or be able to move out of the position due to the head and shoulders being pressed back. The child is also at risk of lateral curvature of the spine, the severely adducted hip is in a vulnerable position for dislocation, the left arm will become fixed in flexion. From this position there is no potential to develop any normal motor activity

Fig. 9.4   Some common patterns of deformity seen in cerebral palsy.

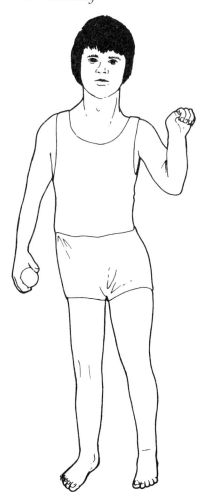

Hemiplegic posture.
The hemiplegic child, not encouraged to weight-bear or use the hemiplegic side, will show release of abnormal postural reflex activity in the form of associated reactions. This can lead to permanent increase of spasticity and common deformities include TA and hamstring tightness (also causing limb length discrepancy) and elbow, wrist and hand flexor contracture

The 'creeping' of the spastic diplegic
The diplegic uses increased flexion in his 'good' arms, the abnormal pulling of the arms into the body bends the head and rounds the back, it also causes increased stiffness of the legs. Continued activity leads to loss of full range of the arms and spine into extension of the thoracic spine. This also compounds adductor and plantar flexion tightness

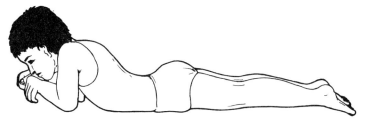

Fig. 9.4 Continued.

In many instances the apparent contracture may not yet be structural and can be reversed by counteracting the pattern of spasticity responsible. For example, an apparent flexor contracture of the knees may still be reversible if extension of hips and spine is achieved to create an environment of posture in which knee extension becomes a possibility. Another example is the use of reflex inhibiting patterns for positioning, for instance, side lying can be used to position a child with ATNR. This facilitates control of the head, as lack of pressure on the back of the head prevents strong retraction of neck and shoulders and also enables the child to get his hands together, where he can see them. Hips can be controlled by placing a cushion between the thighs. Not only does reflex inhibiting posturing help to address the problem of deformity, it also enables a more normal background posture to be created, from which normal movement patterns may be initiated.

Braces and splints should not be used as a matter of course where deformity is impending, but should be carefully tailored to the child's individual needs. Any distal stretch of spastic muscles may cause shift of spasticity to the nearest free joint, as muscles do not act over only one joint. For instance, a wrist extension splint may deal with the extension of the wrist locally, but shunt the spasticity proximally to produce increased flexion and pronation at the elbow, more retraction of the shoulder and possibly increased truncal asymmetry. Hence, in dealing with one problem, others arise which may result in a more severe problem than the original. Although any bracing or splinting used must be very carefully monitored, the calculated use of localized splinting as an aid to treatment can be extremely useful. Leg gaiters may be used to maintain extension of the knees when treating a child in standing, but this should again be carefully monitored to avoid dependency.

Where structural changes of tendons or joints have occurred, or a hip is in danger of dislocating, surgery may be necessary. The physiotherapist has an important role in preparing children for surgery and in their postoperative rehabilitation, so that full use can be made of surgical corrections.

In conclusion, improved motor function involves a holistic approach, which is child-centred. To be successful the physiotherapist needs to be part of a team which is multidisciplinary, forward-looking, closely knit and goal-orientated.

9.5 Principles of orthopaedic surgery in cerebral palsy

Cerebral palsy is a non-progressive disorder of motor function which occurs in early life. However, the manifestations of the disorder may be progressive in nature. The degree of the disability is related to the size and the position of the lesion, and therefore each child has a different degree of involvement.

The role of the orthopaedic surgeon is as part of a multidisciplinary team looking after the child as a whole. There is no place for an orthopaedic surgeon to carry out the occasional orthopaedic procedure. The surgeon is part of the team whose goal is to enable the child to fulfil its potential and the goal for each child is different.

The two major patterns that present different problems to the orthopaedic surgeon are:

1. the child with spasticity;
2. those with disorders of movement, dyskinetic or ataxic.

In the child with spasticity there is an imbalance between muscle activity in flexor and extensor groups; the difference may be one of increased tone and/or different muscle strengths. Imbalance will lead to deformity in the growing child. It may be possible to overcome deformity that is related to posture or increased muscle tone. If there is a difference in true muscle power, however, then the deformity will become fixed. It is often said that in this group the deformity is due to a development of a contracture, but this is a misconception. The contracture develops because strong muscle fails to grow and becomes short.

It is this group of children who may benefit from orthopaedic surgery to correct the deformity and to prevent its recurrence by achieving muscle balance around the joints. By contrast, surgery has little part to play in the management of children with disorders of movement as they rarely develop fixed deformities.

Muscle balance is achieved by either dividing, lengthening or transferring tendons. Muscles can be weakened by crushing the nerves or performing neurectomies. There is little place in young children for bone surgery, but in some cases joint fusions are useful in the older child.

The orthopaedic surgeon has very definite aims in the treatment of the child with cerebral palsy. These are:

1. to improve function;
2. to prevent pain;
3. to improve hygiene;
4. to improve appearance.

To determine what is necessary or possible, or what is required at what time, requires a full functional assessment of the child. It is essential that orthopaedic surgeons are involved early in the management of these children to enable them to perform repeated evaluations of the child's progress and development. The assessment should be carried out in conjunction with the physiotherapist so that the child's progress can be discussed. In this way the development of contractures can be identified early and, with appropriate treatment, prevented.

It is not recommended that the decision regarding treatment is made on the basis of one visit. It is better to see children regularly to gain their confidence, and the confidence of their parents, before deciding on any surgical intervention. The findings on examination of a cooperative child may be totally different from the findings in a child who is upset, frightened or crying, and whose tone is often increased.

The early management of the child with a motor dysfunction is physiotherapy. The role of the physiotherapist is to encourage and help the child in sitting, standing, crawling and, if possible, walking. All joints should be put through a full range of movement to prevent the development of contractures if at all possible. Rigorous stretching of muscles may help them grow and may therefore prevent the occurrence of deformities of joints. Orthoses and splints can be used to maintain the correct position of joints at the time of rest. At this early stage, orthoses are often valuable in maintaining the position of joints when early weight-bearing is attempted. The application of plaster casts to the feet has been shown to help reduce the tone in triceps surae in many children. Orthopaedic surgery is required when physiotherapy has been unable to prevent joint deformity by contractures in muscles.

The timing of any surgical intervention is critical. In some instances it may be considered to be quite urgent, while in other cases operations should be designed to fit in with the child's total management. Every effort should be made to fit in with school and physiotherapy programmes, and any family commitments. If more than one operation is required, if at all possible these should be carried out under the same anaesthetic. This will remove the problem of repeated hospital admissions, periods of immobilization and rehabilitation. Planning the type of surgery to be undertaken may be helped by the use of electromyography and gait analysis studies. These may be of value in some children with diplegia and hemiplegia, but to undergo these investigations the child must be functioning well intellectually and be willing to cooperate. Some of the information gained in these analyses may be difficult to interpret.

Surgery should be delayed as long as possible in the child's management because, as the child develops, there may be spontaneous improvement. Indeed suggestions have been made that children with diplegia should not undergo surgery before the age of 7.

The aims of surgery should be stressed to the family, who must be aware of what it is hoped to achieve; after the operation the child still has cerebral palsy, and the parents will need to be aware of this. The parents and carers of the child should be cognisant of the requirements of the child during the postoperative period, and what will be required of them. The child should return to his physiotherapist after surgery, and any splints or orthosis that will be required in the postoperative phase should be obtained, if at all possible, prior to the surgical event or soon after. It is essential that regular physiotherapy is commenced after surgery to maintain the corrected joint range following any operative procedure.

What surgery has to offer is best divided into three separate areas.

(a)   Lower limbs

Contractures produce malalignment of the weight-bearing joints. The goal in orthopaedic surgery is to realign the weight-bearing joints and to achieve muscle balance around the joints, so that further deformity does not develop. This gives the child a stable platform on which to walk. Correction of deformity also reduces the energy expenditure which is required to walk. Once correct position is achieved, orthosis or splints can help maintain this position.

The aim with this group of patients is to improve their function. However, in a number of children with total body involvement who will not walk, surgery is also indicated. We know that these children often have very tight abductors and hip flexors, and this leads to dislocation. Dislocation of the hip is a painful experience, and by judicious surgery of an adductor and flexor release, dislocation in the child with total body involvement can be prevented. Therefore surgery should not be denied to these children because of their severe involvement, because the pain of a dislocated hip increases the tone and compounds their condition. In addition, obtaining a good abduction range helps cleaning and perineal toilet of these children.

Even if a child is not going to walk, deformity of the feet can be a significant problem. Simple surgery can maintain the foot in a position in which it is possible to obtain footwear.

(b)   Upper limbs

There is a small percentage of hemiplegic children with deformity of the upper limb, in whom surgery can be of value to improve function. Although, in the vast majority of hemiplegic children, the function will not be improved by surgery, a significant proportion of these children need not be denied any operative intervention. Most hemiplegic children attend normal school and have normal intellectual performance, but may experience considerable teasing by their peers because of a deformity of a flexed elbow and a flexed wrist. Simple surgical measures can give them a straight arm which they can hide in a pocket and this certainly leads to less embarrassment. Another bonus of straightening out the arm is that it makes dressing significantly easier.

In the quadriplegic child who has both arms involved, with the advent of computers and computer keyboards, surgery has a great part to play. Being unable to speak and having poor hand function, communication for these children is exceptionally difficult. To straighten out a hand so that one finger can work a keyboard can make a significant difference to the environment of these children.

Severely involved children who have clenched fingers may suffer from nails cutting into the palm. This becomes increasingly painful, cleaning of the hand is difficult and the skin often becomes lacerated. Simple tendon divisions can straighten out the hand and relieve these symptoms.

(c) Spine

A number of children develop scoliosis, often a long 'C' curve. The majority of these malformations are postural, and for the most part can be controlled by special seating arrangements, adaptations to wheelchairs, or braces. However, if all these adaptations fail to control the development of the scoliosis, then there is a place for surgery. A child with significant scoliosis will have limitation of respiratory function. If the curve leads to decompensation of the spine, the child will fall to one side whilst sitting, and will effectively defunction one hand.

10   *Seating*

A child learns to hold the head up, sit with a straight back and move in and out of a sitting position within the first year of life (Table 10.1). Normal muscle tone and the developmental of normal postural reflexes provide the foundation upon which all these sitting skills develop.

The child with cerebral palsy generally has abnormal muscle tone and often retains primitive reflexes and develops disruptive pathological reflexes. These reflexes interfere with normal movement and also hinder the development of the normal righting and equilibrium reactions that promote balance and stability. Independent sitting for a child with cerebral palsy can therefore become a very complex task to master.

The provision of good postural seating is vital, not only to enable the child to view his environment, but more importantly to allow her the opportunity to develop her sitting ability.

The child with cerebral palsy spends a long time sitting, particularly when at school, and only receives comparatively short periods of active therapy. Seating equipment, therefore, must complement and reinforce the therapeutic principles on which the child's treatment is based.

10.1   The aims of good postural seating

1. To establish a stable sitting position: by positioning the pelvis in a neutral position and allowing weight to be taken through the ischial tuberosities.
2. To reduce abnormal reflex activity: by introducing reflex inhibiting postures, and thereby increasing the possibility of normal movement.
3. To prevent/correct postural deformity: if postural deformity is not corrected it will become fixed. Uncorrected pelvic obliquity causes a compensatory scoliosis and may lead to hip dislocation. Uncorrected sacral sitting can cause compensatory thoracic kyphosis. All these deformities can be limited, if not avoided altogether, with good

Table 10.1 Development of sitting ability

1 month	3 months	6 months	9 months	12 months	18 months
Marked head lag in pull-to-sit. Held in sitting, head falls forward.	Slight head lag in pull-to-sit. When held in sitting, holds back straight, except in lumbar region, with head erect for short periods then drops it forwards.	Sits with support, able to turn head from side to side. Head firmly erect and straight back. May sit alone momentarily.	Sits with good control for 10–15 minutes. Able to reach forward and to sit without losing balance. Pulls self to standing.	Sits well for indefinite periods of time. Able to attain sitting position from lying. Able to prop backwards and turn to play.	Able to walk to and seat self in small chair.

Adapted from Sheridan (1975).

postural seating used in conjunction with appropriate and timely surgical intervention.

4. To maximize upper limb function: to facilitate the development of hand–eye coordination and fine manipulation. This can in turn promote independence in self-care activities, such as self-feeding.

10.1.1 SEAT ORIENTATION – UPRIGHT VERSUS RECLINED

It is often the assumption that children who are unable to sit well in an upright chair (usually because of inadequate or inappropriate support), would be better positioned if the chair were reclined. However, research suggests this theory is incorrect.

Nwaobi (1987) has studied the effect of seating orientation on the child with cerebral palsy and found that tonic muscle activity measured by electromyography was less in the upright position than the reclined, i.e. abnormal reflexes were reduced by upright sitting. Also the orientation of the body in space was found to affect upper limb function, the highest level of performance being recorded in the upright position.

Pauline Pope, in her study of severely disabled adults, concluded that the reclined position is undesirable where instability of trunk and pelvis is a problem. It encourages the trunk to slide down the chair, resulting in a slouched posture and increasing the risk of tissue damage (Pope, 1985a).

Observation of normal development indicates the reclined position is not conducive to the development of sitting ability, as infants learn to sit from a position of forward prop, that is, with their trunk weight well forward over their sitting base. A child with cerebral palsy who has not yet learnt to forward prop will be unable to develop this ability from a position of recline as it requires mature postural reactions to sit up from this position.

10.1.2 ASSESSMENT

The assessment procedure for seating should take account of the following points. Firstly, it is necessary to examine the reasons why a new chair is required. For example, the child may have outgrown a present chair or physical abilities may have changed such that the present chair may provide too much or too little support or cause pressure trauma. Secondly, the function of the new chair should be considered. It may be required to facilitate specific functions such as operating a wheelchair or self-feeding. Accordingly it may need to adjust to table height to enable the child to eat with the family or may have to be used as an insert for a wheelchair. Finally, and most importantly, the child's abilities must be considered. The child should not merely be observed in sitting, but also in the positions of lying, supine, prone and side lying, pull-to-sit, long sitting, sitting on a flat box, sitting on a ramped cushion and in standing (Mulcahy *et al.*, 1988).

In all positions the following should be noted:

1. asymmetry;
2. weight distribution;
3. alignment of the pelvis and its position relative to the trunk;
4. any present or potential deformities and contractures, particularly at hips, knees, ankles and spine;
5. support required for the child to conform and maintain position;
6. child's ability to move within positions and in and out of position.

10.1.3   CHOOSING THE RIGHT TYPE OF CHAIR

The information gained through assessment should be recorded to give a baseline of the child's ability. This can then be used as a basis for the prescription of seats.

Mulcahy *et al.* (1988) have developed principles to describe 'seven levels of sitting ability' (Table 10.2, Fig. 10.1).

10.2   A closer look at supportive chairs

10.2.1   UPRIGHT CHAIRS

There are now a number of upright, right-angled chairs available that are specifically designed to seat children with cerebral palsy. It is not appropriate to describe each 'make' of chair, with its advantages and disadvantages, since new designs and modifications are continuously evolving. It is more helpful to discuss in greater detail the different features of an upright chair which have already been mentioned (Table 10.2).

10.2.2   PELVIC SUPPORT

(a)   Ramped cushion

It has been assumed for some time that sitting a child in an upright, right-angled chair will automatically position the hips and knees at a 90° angle. However, anthropometric measurements and clinical

Table 10.2 Assessment of sitting ability used as a basis for the prescription of a suitable seat

Level of sitting ability*	Purpose of seat	Type of seat suitable
1. Unplaceable: child cannot be easily placed into a sitting position, i.e. she cannot anchor her bottom or dissociate her upper trunk.	– to provide totally supportive position. Emphasis on postural fixation to stabilize pelvis. – alternative positions important, e.g. side lying, prone standing.	(i) Right-angled seat with control to pelvis using ramped cushion, sacral pad, pelvic strap and knee blocks. Foot support, lateral trunk support, head support, and chest strap/pad as appropriate. An upright position should be introduced as soon as possible, e.g. Chailey Adaptor seat, James Lecky Design chair (NB: has sacral roll not pad). (ii) If the child has severe fixed deformities of spine and/or hips a more intimately contoured chair may need to be considered. A child not tolerating an upright position may need a chair with reclining facilities, e.g. Chailey moulded seat, Derby moulded seat, Matrix seat. (iii) An alternative seating position for part of the day could be considered as a different means of introducing upright sitting, such as stabilizing pelvis on saddle type seat, with trunk supported anterior to the sitting base, e.g. straddle seat (Stewart and McQuilton, 1987).

2. Placeable but *cannot maintain* position independently.	– to provide very supportive symmetrical position which stabilizes pelvis and encourages upright sitting.	(i) Very supportive, upright, right-angled chair which stabilizes pelvis using ramped cushion, sacral pad and pelvic strap, also incorporating knee block or pommel. Lateral trunk support and chest strap/pad will promote symmetry and security. A forward work position can be encouraged by the use of a tray with grab bar. (ii) Alternative forward sitting position to promote upper limb function, e.g. Jenx prone chair.
3. Maintain position but *unable to move*, i.e. can just maintain balance with both hands used for support.	– to provide sufficient support to maintain sitting balance and so free hands for play and activities of daily living.	Upright, right-angled chair with control to pelvis as in level 2. Gradual reduction of lateral and head support as sitting ability improves. For example, upright chair made of plywood with padding, Jenx chair, Rifton chair.
4. Maintain position, move within base only, i.e. confidently moves forward over base but unable to raise arms to shoulder, or lean far to the side before losing balance.	– to provide stable base which will encourage development of straight back posture. The chair should allow forward prop position and free upper limbs for use.	Upright, right-angled seat with control to pelvis as in level 2. Some lateral support and/or armrests which can be reduced or removed as ability improves. Use of pommel will increase width of sitting base.
5. Maintain position, move outside base, i.e. reaches and regains balance.	– to provide stable base but allow weight transfer laterally.	Upright, right-angled seat with ramped cushion. Feet should be flat on floor if possible, to encourage child to reach out of base. A tray or table at correct height will increase stability. Arm rest should be removable. Mainly used for security (e.g. if chair used in transit).

Table 10.2 *(continued)*

Level of sitting ability*	*Purpose of seat*	*Type of seat suitable*
6. Move out of position but cannot retain or attain sitting.	– to provide stable base on which to encourage development of a more mature sitting posture.	Upright, right-angled chair which allows feet to be placed flat on floor to allow transfer.
		Table at appropriate height.
		Child must be able to undo any security straps if she is to be independent in transfers.
7. Attain position (probably still learning to walk independently).	– to provide stable, comfortable base.	Stable, upright chair with backrest to provide resting position.
		Child needs to be able to do and undo any security straps.
		Work table at suitable height.
		For example, simple wooden chair at correct height and correct hip to knee dimensions.

Adapted from Mulcahy and Pountney, 'Prescription of seats by assessment of sitting ability' (Mulcahy, Pountney *et al.*, 1988).
*Numbers correspond to levels of ability as depicted in Fig. 10.1

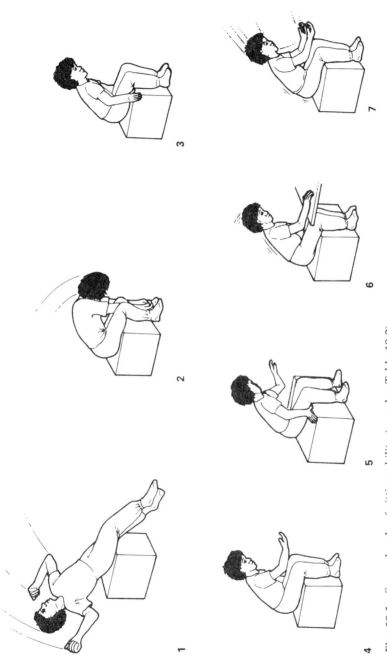

Fig. 10.1 Seven levels of sitting ability (see also Table 10.2).

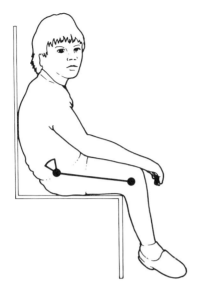
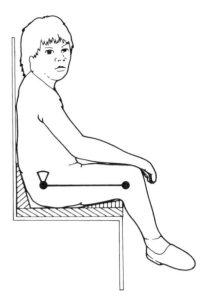

Fig. 10.2 Note posterior tilt of pelvis and downward sloping femur.

Fig. 10.3 Use of ramped cushion and sacral pad to position femur in horizontal plane and to stabilize pelvis.

observations have shown that sitting on a horizontal surface actually maintains the femur in a downward sloping angle, which leads the pelvis to tilt posteriorly and causes the child to sit sacrally (Fig. 10.2).

A cushion ramped at a 15° angle will accommodate the thigh and position the femur in a horizontal plane (Fig. 10.3). The cushion should begin to angle upwards 1–2 cm anterior to the gluteal crease and continue to the popliteal fossa leaving the area under the buttocks flat so that weight is taken through the ischial tuberosities (Fig. 10.4) (Mulcahy and Pountney, 1987).

(b)   Sacral pad

The sacral pad is designed to maintain the pelvis in an anterior/neutral tilt and so facilitate the development of a more upright posture (Fig. 10.3). It should be positioned at the base of the child's backrest, at a 90° angle to the base seat. The pad should be made of firm foam approximately 2 cm thick and angled from the height of the lumbosacral junction (L5/SI) (Fig. 10.4) (Mulcahy and Pountney, 1986).

The sacral pad is designed to be used in conjunction with a ramped cushion and pelvic strap.

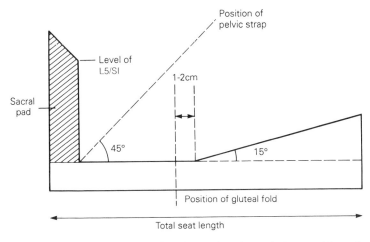

Fig. 10.4 Cross-section of ramped cushion showing relative position of sacral pad and pelvic strap (Mulcahy and Pountney, 1986, 1987).

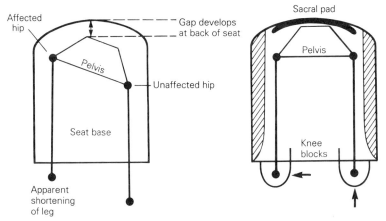

Fig. 10.5 Showing windswept hips. Note rotation of pelvis allowing gap to develop at back of chair.

Fig. 10.6 Showing effect of knee blocks to reverse postural windsweeping of hips. Arrows indicate direction of force.

(c)   Pelvic strap

To be effective the strap should pass anterior to the pelvis at a 45° angle to the base of the seat (Fig. 10.4).

(d)   Knee block

A knee block can be used in addition to the above to provide even greater control to the pelvis. It can also be an effective means of controlling windswept hips. Force is applied anteriorly to the unaffected hip via the distal end of the femur and the tibial tuberosity, which causes the pelvis to derotate and so abduct the affected hip (Figs 10.5 and 10.6).

It is essential that the knee block is bilateral, to ensure the corrective force does not cause the pelvis to overcompensate by rotating in the opposite direction to overadduct the originally unaffected hip.

(e)   Pommel/adduction block

A pommel is usually wedge-shaped and is positioned between the medial surfaces of the thighs (Fig. 10.7). It encourages hip abduction, which provides a wider sitting base, inhibits extensor spasm and reduces the risk of hip dislocation.

10.2.3   THORACIC AND HEAD SUPPORT

(a)   Lateral trunk support

Supports should align with chest contours and maintain the trunk and spine in midline (Figs 10.7 and 10.8). They should not interfere with upper limb function.

(b)   Chest pad/strap

The use of a chest pad or strap is usually more effective than shoulder straps for maintaining the trunk in an upright position, particularly for children with truncal hypotonia.

(c)   Head support

A head rest extension fitted to the chair may provide sufficient support. If the child's head persistently drops to the side, lateral head supports, or a 'banana' pillow, could be introduced, especially to support the head at mealtimes (Fig. 10.8). Lateral supports should be removed as soon as possible to encourage independent head control. If the head persistently drops forward, reclining the chair is occasionally the only option, with the gradual introduction of a more upright position over time. An alternative forward leaning position used for

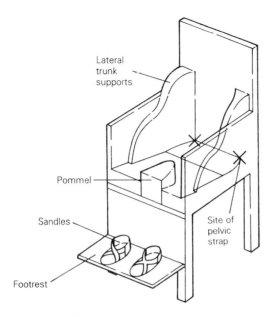

Fig. 10.7   A pommel.

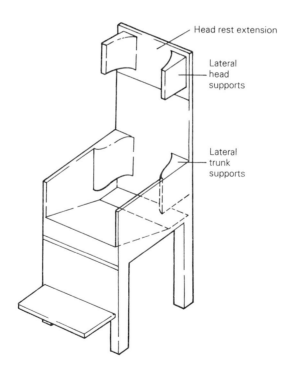

Fig. 10.8   Lateral trunk and head supports.

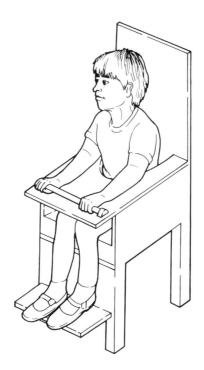

Fig. 10.9 A tray.

short periods of the day, e.g. prone standing, may also improve head control.

10.2.4 ADDITIONAL STABILITY FEATURES

(a) Tray

A tray positioned at elbow height or slightly higher will provide extra stability and encourage forward propping (Fig. 10.9).

(b) Grab bar

A grab bar attached to the tray further increases stability, particularly if used with arm gaiters (Fig. 10.9).

(c) Foot rests and sandles

It is important that knees and ankles are positioned at a 90° angle. Children with sitting ability of level 4 or less (see Table 10.2) should all be sat on chairs with an adjustable height foot rest. Extra stability can

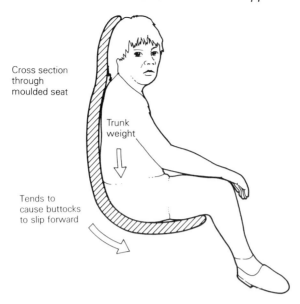

Cross section
through
moulded seat

Trunk
weight

Tends to
cause buttocks
to slip forward

Fig. 10.10 Disadvantages of a moulded seat.

be provided by the use of sandles to hold the feet and ankles in the
desired position (Fig. 10.7).

10.2.5 FORWARD LEANING SEATS

These chairs are primarily designed to seat the child with cerebral palsy
during functional therapy. They are based on the principle that
forward leaning brings the centre of gravity in the upper trunk anterior
to the pelvis, thus reducing the degree of lumbosacral flexion
(Brunswic, 1984), reducing the effort required to bring the upper limbs
into a position of function, and improving the child's upright sitting
posture by causing the extensor muscles of the back and neck to
counteract gravity (Myhr and von Wendt, 1991).

The chairs usually seat the children in a similar position to that
obtained on horseback. Reducing hip flexion and tilting the pelvis
forward tends to reduce reflexive extensor activity, thereby promoting
upper limb function (Stewart and McQuilton, 1987).

10.2.6 INTIMATELY CONTOURED SEATS

These seats are fitted and made up professionally for individual
children. Examples include the Derby moulded seat, Chailey moulded

seat and Matrix. (NB: The Matrix seat is the only seating system in this group which can be significantly adapted to allow for growth or physical changes in the child's abilities.)

Over the past few years, moulded seats have been widely prescribed for children with a low level of sitting ability. They were believed to give good postural support and relief of pressure by distributing it over a larger surface area. Recently the disadvantages of moulded seating have been realized (Stewart and McQuilton, 1987; Mulcahy *et al.*, 1988).

The base of the moulded seat is contoured to the shape of the buttocks. As the centre of gravity is posterior to the sitting base, the weight of the trunk causes the body to slip down the chair. This in turn causes the pelvis to tilt backwards adapting to the round contours of the base, thus giving rise to sacral sitting and the possible development of tissue trauma (Fig. 10.10).

However, the moulded seat continues to be useful for children with severe fixed deformities that cannot be suitably accommodated by 'ready-made' chairs.

11 *Eating and drinking*

11.1 Assessment

This section discusses the child's physical control of oral patterns of movement for eating and drinking. Morris and Klein (1987) provides more detailed discussion of feeding difficulties and therapeutic procedures.

Eating and drinking behaviour can be assessed in terms of:

1. adequacy of
   (a) nutrition
   (b) efficiency of feeding patterns
   (c) tolerance
   (d) technique;
2. social implications for
   (a) the family
   (b) the child
   (c) the professionals.

11.1.1 ADEQUACY

(a) Nutrition

One of the most urgent reasons for attempting to modify a child's eating or drinking behaviour is concern over the adequacy of his nutritional and dietary intake. Concern about nutrition may arise for a number of reasons: food and liquid intake may be insufficient for requirements (diet may be poorly balanced with associated health implications); vomiting may cause loss of the food already taken; there may be absorption problems and failure to thrive despite apparently adequate intake; or the carer's perception of the child's nutritional state or needs may be at odds with the professional opinion.

A thorough assessment of intake and loss will need to be made in conjunction with a dietitian and a paediatrician. This is particularly important when reassurance or evidence is required by the carer that nutrition is adequate. A carer who has a sick or poorly nourished child may not willingly try new ideas if there is a possibility that the child's health may further be compromised even in the short term. If nutrition or dietary needs are inadequate, then the dietitian is often able to advise on food supplementation or adaptation appropriate to the child. The knowledge that nutrition is adequate can greatly alleviate tensions experienced during mealtimes and facilitate a more relaxed approach to intervention.

A child who has been nasogastrically fed can present a particular problem for parents and professionals when a transfer to oral feeding is considered. Where immaturity or inadequacy of oral feeding patterns have been the main reasons for nasogastric feeding, the child is likely to have received adequate and reasonably struggle-free intake from the tube. Initially, oral feeding will often involve struggle and less fluid/liquid intake. Care needs to be taken, therefore, to assess nutritional needs, the child's oral competence and the carer's attitudes, so that a planned transition to oral feeds can be made with appropriate monitoring and counselling for carers.

(b)   Efficiency

(i) Speed   A major measurable indicator of the efficiency of the child's eating skills is the speed with which he takes his food (the length of time taken for the meal). Although 'average' lengths of time for meals are not available (because of the vast variation in what constitutes a mealtime), most carers recognize when meals go on for an inordinate length of time, or when the portion fails to diminish in size substantially with the passing of time. The child who eats quickly when presented with 'easy to tackle' foods may nevertheless have eating problems with more difficult foods.

An assessment of mealtime length and the amount and type of food taken will not only supply information but also will reflect the stresses upon the carer and child at mealtimes. If the meal is protracted, the child may become tired and uninterested, his meal may become unappetizing and, if one meal runs into the next, he may not receive the hunger/full signals to rekindle his interest in food. The carer, faced with a never ending cycle of unrewarding mealtimes, can soon become exhausted. In frustration and an attempt to speed things up, carers often use techniques and approaches such as tipping the child back, presenting larger spoonfuls and so on, which can exacerbate existing problems and cause new ones.

(ii) Oral skills   An assessment must include the following.

1. Oral structure – e.g. dentition, enlarged tonsils and adenoids, malocclusion, cleft palate, or any structural problem which could affect eating or drinking.

2. Eating and drinking patterns, e.g. suckling, chewing, biting, swallowing. This is necessary to assess the developmental level achieved by the child for tackling different foods. Such an assessment may necessitate procedures such as videofluoroscopy or nasendoscopy, in which case the child and carer need to be adequately prepared for these intrusive procedures.
3. Movement – assesses the relationships existing between the child's tone, posture, movement and reflexes, and their interactions in differing circumstances, e.g. feeding reflexes may vary in terms of stimulus and strength of response. This will affect tone, posture and movement differently so that a potentially helpful reflex may hinder feeding under certain circumstances or vice versa.

This assessment should show how much can be expected of the child and the order in which goals are set.

4. Breathing – in association with eating and drinking. There is a danger of aspiration, i.e. taking food or liquid into the lungs, and this should be fully investigated at the onset of eating and drinking therapy.

Assessment is best carried out by speech therapist, physiotherapist and occupational therapist, with the carer, over the course of at least one meal with a variety of foods (when appropriate). It may be necessary for the professional personally to attempt some feeding to obtain kinaesthetic feedback. When such 'taking over' is necessary the professional may achieve more success than the carer, who will need appropriate support and explanation to avoid feelings of inadequacy.

(c) Tolerance

Children with eating and drinking problems frequently show poor tolerance of the mealtime and are often deemed naughty, faddy and manipulative. They may appear to dislike the feeding routine, utensils used and the type and temperature of food given, either intermittently or during the meal. Intolerance shows itself in general behaviours like turning away, refusing to eat, crying – some young babies can become totally inert when overstressed – and in more specific food/utensil behaviours by grimacing, gagging and vomiting. A thorough assessment of adequacy of oral sensitivity to taste, texture, temperature and consistency of the food and utensils given must be made, since many children with cerebral palsy have marked oral hypersensitivity. Where appropriate, an investigation may need to be made to identify food allergies etc.

Difficulty at mealtimes can, of course, also be behavioural. The feeding team will need to make a careful assessment of all the factors influencing the child's behaviour and considerable care should be taken to avoid such confrontational labels as 'naughty child' or 'bad mother'. Mealtime issues are very common throughout childhood and into adulthood, and are not confined to families where there is a child with a disability. They can become abnormally highlighted just because the child has a disability, whereas with another child they might be taken as a very normal part of growing up and exerting influence!

(d)   Technique

1. Position: the adequacy of the carer's techniques in positioning a child for eating and in presenting the food to him can greatly influence the efficiency with which the child can eat. An approach to positioning which angles the child's head and neck in such a way that food loss is reduced and gravity helps it down may well result in cleaner eating. However, it is likely also to increase the child's chances of choking and prevent him learning to control the food orally himself. Patterns of feeding are being established and re-inforced which will contribute to his continuing to be reliant upon others to feed him and on eating an unexciting soft diet. An ade-quate assessment of position of both child and carer is vital since it is the key point for any remedial programme devised.

2. Utensils: there is a wide variety of teats, spoons and cups available. Any assessment should include details of which utensils are used to feed the child, e.g. is a deep bowled spoon or a small flat one used, is the child given a large teat with a small hole or a small teat with a large hole, is the teat straight or cherry topped, or orthodontic, etc.?

3. Texture: the assessor needs to know with what sort of food is presented to the child – smooth, thick, runny, lumpy, mashed, etc.

4. Taste: it is important to assess the types of food offered to the child and whether the child seems to prefer sweet or savoury, strong flavours or bland.

5. Carer's use of utensils: the carer's choice of utensils, speed of pre-sentation, method of food preparation, amount presented and ways of manipulating utensils in the child's mouth will greatly influence what type of food the child can manage, the maturity of feeding patterns he can achieve and how much he can actively participate in the mealtime. The speech therapist's assessment must, therefore, include a detailed assessment of how and with what the child is fed. The therapist will need to evaluate the likely effect of utensils and technique on the child's feeding pattern, and hypotheses will need to be tested with other utensils, food or feeding techniques. Again, there is a risk of upsetting the mother–child relationship, especially

if the new utensils/techniques do improve the situation. Sensitive assessment involving parent and professionals discovering new techniques for the child *together* is vital to parental self-esteem and self-confidence.

11.1.2 SOCIAL IMPLICATION

(a) For the family

To most new parents, the baby's uncanny ability to wake for food at the mother's mealtimes, no matter how irregular, is at best amusing and at worst frustrating. When a child has eating problems, the frustration is considerably increased by feelings of inadequacy, guilt at neglecting the rest of the family, and fears for the child's well-being.

As the baby grows older, instead of becoming less dependent on adult involvement, he may need more adult time to help him finish his meal. As a result of this, the carer, often the mother, and the child may be isolated from the rest of the family, resulting in considerable increase in stress. It is important to assess the family's attitude towards mealtimes: have they adapted themselves to the child to the disadvantage of their own well-being and family life? Do they see any alternatives to the way in which mealtimes are conducted? What do they see as the cause of the problem? For example: 'If he could chew, it would help a lot'; 'He is so slow, if we could speed him up, it would help.'

If the child is hospitalized for any length of time, or attends a day centre, day nursery or school, he may be fed by a variety of other people. The therapists should be aware of possible inconsistencies in the handling of the child at mealtimes, and try, by the use of diagrams and eating and drinking guidelines, to ensure consistency of approach.

(b) For the child

Given the stress that may surround mealtimes, the child may not be getting the social stimulation usually available to children at this time. The child may be all too aware of the tensions aroused in others at mealtimes and find this a negative experience. Physical discomfort, and therefore defensiveness, may result from early incoordination and current feeding difficulties and, in consequence, instead of being pleasant social occasions, mealtimes may be unpleasant and distressing for the child.

In a child who is fairly severely affected physically, choosing what to eat or whether to eat at all may be one of the only areas in his life where he has significant control. He may find the tension and agitation he can produce in his carer quite entertaining and, especially if he has learned to be orally defensive, a serious behaviour problem can result. The involvement of a clinical psychologist is invaluable here.

11.2   Therapy for eating and drinking

Therapy for eating and drinking problems is complex, and the fine details will depend on the nature of the child's problem and the interaction between physical and behavioural aspects and the stage of therapy at the time. Warner (1981) and Morris and Klein (1987) discuss feeding therapy in considerable detail: here the major issues will be outlined.

Mention has already been made elsewhere of the danger of invading the parent–child dyad during therapy. Mealtimes are particularly vulnerable to invasion, especially as the parents may be feeling inadequate in their difficulties in feeding their child. Suggestions, therefore, should be made with care and with respect for the parent–child relationship.

11.2.1   POSITION

A suitable feeding position should be found through experimentation. If the child has a tendency to be extended or constantly moving, it is important to find a position where the head can be upright by offering support for the base of the head without pushing the head forward. The hips and knees should be flexed, and the head and shoulders kept forward.

Children who are mainly flexed or who are floppy will need a position which helps them keep their head from flopping forward or back. The head can be supported in a very slightly reclining seat or by the carer controlling the head from the side.

11.2.2   SENSITIVITY

The child may show hyper- or hyposensitivity. Both can affect eating efficiency. If the child is showing oral hypersensitivity it is important to encourage carers to spend time before each meal desensitizing the face and mouth. This is done by firm tapping or stroking on the face, moving from the forehead and near to the ears, in and down towards the nose and mouth and ending with the mouth by stroking and tapping inside, including the gums in the front of the mouth, and towards the back teeth. The child should also be encouraged to mouth toys and his own fingers as much as possible.

Where a child is showing hyposensitivity, there may be a need for oral sensitization, i.e. bringing through the baby's primary reflexes. Oral stimulation may also be necessary to identify problems in 'practice sessions', not using real food.

11.2.3   UTENSILS

The size, shape and flow of the teat will depend on the individual child's problem. For example, a child who has not yet developed a suckling reflex may need a soft straight teat which reaches to the back of the tongue to stimulate suckling.

When weaning, spoons should be narrow and not have a deep bowl, which will discourage a child from pulling food off the spoon with his top lip. The spoon should be of plastic rather than metal as, if the child has a bite reflex, he is less likely to damage his teeth or hurt his gums. It is sometimes necessary to put food into a child's mouth with fingers.

11.2.4   TASTE

It is important to encourage the child to take a variety of different tastes. However, if the child prefers sweet food to savoury, for example, it is not advisable to introduce savoury food at the same time as introducing a new technique for feeding, e.g. finger feeding or a very different texture.

Some tastes will stimulate suckling, e.g. sugar, vinegar used in small amounts, etc. The type of texture used will depend on the stage the child is at, and the programme of therapy. Some textures may cause a gag reflex in a sensitive child, e.g. mashed potato, peas, baked beans, and can be difficult for a child to deal with. Some baby foods and soups consist of slightly thickened liquid with lumps of vegetable or meat. This texture can be very difficult for the child to deal with. The two very different textures require different methods, drinking the liquid and squashing lumps, and the child may not be able to cope with drinking a liquid having selected the lumps for subsequent squashing. For introducing lumpy food, a progressively thicker but fairly smooth texture is required.

11.2.5   TECHNIQUE

When encouraging suckling, having established the position and experimented with teats to find the one that suits the child best, the child can be encouraged to suckle by stimulation of reflexes as he has the bottle in his mouth. If necessary, his jaw should be held forward by the thumb during feeding.

When introducing the child to solid food, he must be encouraged away from the suckling pattern, which is a backwards and forwards movement of the tongue, to a chewing pattern, which includes an up and down movement and a side to side movement. If the food is presented in the centre of the child's mouth, suckling may well continue, but if the food is presented to either side of the child's mouth, so that it is dropped between the child's gums using a small narrow spoon, the chewing reflex may be stimulated by the food on the gums. Under these circumstances the child will have more opportunity to move the food around his mouth before he moves it to the centre and swallows it, and the risk of gagging is reduced. The food can be presented to the mouth by spoon or by the fingers using small lumps of potato, carrot, cheese, fish or any food which will 'collapse' easily in the mouth, but which is firm enough to push between the child's cheek and teeth. When progressing from smooth food to lumpy food, this is best done gradually, presenting the child with a few lumps at the beginning of the meal, and then completing the meal with his usual texture and gradually increasing the number of lumps.

11.2.6   BEHAVIOUR

Given bad early experiences, due to sensitivity and lack of coordination, and possibly the realization that he can control the environment to some extent through refusing to eat, or eating only certain foods, behaviour problems can occur in children with feeding difficulties. Any programme should be devised in conjunction with the psychologists and the dietitian. The dietitian will be able to ensure that the child has adequate nutrition for his needs through supplements, thereby relieving some of the tension felt by the parents. The clinical psychologist will be able to look at the feeding patterns that the family have developed, and advise on how these patterns may be adapted. The speech therapist's role is to advise on the child's physical ability to deal with the food he is being offered.

11.2.7   DRINKING

When moving their child from a bottle to a cup, many parents use trainer beakers with a nozzle. These nozzles, whilst being convenient for the child in avoiding spillage, in fact encourage the same suckling patterns as a bottle. The most useful are feeder cups with a short broad nozzle, which tend to encourage slightly different patterns. A Doidy cup is useful as the extended lip helps to flatten the tongue and discourage suckling, and it is possible to see how much liquid is going into the child's mouth, and whether or not his lip has touched the liquid to draw it in.

Behaviour problems may occur with drinking, as liquid is much more difficult to control than solids, and children feel vulnerable, especially if in the past their airway has been compromised.

12   *Cognitive abilities*

Children with cerebral palsy have a substantially increased risk of showing some degree of cognitive impairment (Nielson, 1971; Cruikshank *et al.*, 1976). These learning difficulties may range from severe global intellectual retardation affecting all areas of the child's life, through to mild or specific learning difficulties, whose only impact is in their influence on aspects of the child's educational progress. While as a group only approximately one-third of children with cerebral palsy will function within the average range intellectually (Stephen and Hawks, 1974), learning difficulty is not an inevitable accompaniment of the motor disabilities of cerebral palsy. Also, while in cerebral palsy children with spastic quadriplegia are more likely to have learning difficulties, there is not a simple relationship between the degree of physical disability and the degree of cognitive impairment. Some children with a hemiplegia may also have serious learning difficulties, while occasionally individuals with severe and complex physical impairments can demonstrate significant intellectual strengths if enabled to do so. This is perhaps well illustrated by Christy Nolan (Nolan, 1981), whose abilities in writing poetry emerged after he was enabled to communicate.

12.1   Factors affecting learning

12.1.1   CNS FACTORS

The cognitive impairments of cerebral palsy are accounted for almost entirely by the central nervous system (CNS) aetiology of the motor deficits. Learning difficulties are largely associated with rather than secondary to physical disabilities. Studies of the cognitive functioning of children with spina bifida (Lorber, 1971; Spain, 1974) have shown that intellectual impairment in these children is related to CNS involvement evidenced by the presence of hydrocephalus rather than to the degree of physical disability. Similarly studies of children with motor

disabilities consequent on thalidomide have failed to show any relationship between degree of physical disability and intelligence (Decarie,
1969).

12.1.2 PSYCHOSOCIAL FACTORS

While neurological dysfunction may make the largest contribution
to the learning difficulties of children with cerebral palsy, there are
indications of cognitive defects in young children whose motor disabilities are not related to central nervous system damage (Decarie,
1969; Wasserman *et al.*, 1985). Decarie explained the lower than
average score of her group of thalidomide children in terms of environmental factors, in that there was a relationship in her sample
between length of time in hospital or institutions and cognitive ability.
In the study carried out by Wasserman *et al.* (1985), different styles of
maternal interaction were found for physically handicapped versus
normal toddlers. These studies are consistent with a transactional
perspective (Sameroff and Chandler, 1975) in suggesting that motor
impairments may affect the child's psychosocial environment in such a
way as to lead to cognitive deficits. For the child with cerebral palsy
who also has intrinsic learning difficulties, the contribution of potential
secondary environmentally based effects on her cognitive development
should not be ignored.

12.1.3 LEARNING THROUGH ACTION

Most studies of the cognitive development of children with physical
handicaps including cerebral palsy make use of measures of global
cognitive functioning, i.e. the intelligence test. The difficulties in using
and interpreting psychometric tests with this population of children
will be discussed later, but even if they have adequate validity and
reliability in use, such measures give little information as to qualitative
aspects of the child's cognitive development, being concerned rather
crudely with product rather than process. One question which has
been posed is to what extent active exploration of the environment is
important for the learning of specific concepts within the usual time
scale. The child's active exploration of his environment appears particularly important in Piaget's (1953) sensori-motor stage, where he
holds that in the first two years infants construct their beliefs about
objects through actively manipulating the environment. Concepts such
as object permanence would therefore be markedly delayed in children
with motor impairments who were not able to be active within their
environment. However, both Decarie (1969) and Kopp and Shaperman
(1973) demonstrated age-appropriate emergence of this concept in chil-

dren who had had no ability to manipulate objects or to be independently mobile. Such achievements in these children suggest that concepts such as object permanence can be acquired in the absence of active manipulation of material. Kagan (1970) and Zelazo (1979) propose that infants are capable of developing perceptual and conceptual structures through observation alone and are therefore able to receive sensory information, store and integrate it at a central level without the necessity of physical participation in the event or overt motoric manipulation.

While these studies involving children with physical handicaps, and work in the field of early developmental psychology (Osofsky, 1979; Wolman, 1982) indicate that motor actions are not a prerequisite for all kinds of learning, this cannot be taken to imply that cognitive development is completely independent of motor development. Kagan (1970) considers that motor skills may indeed be important for some aspects of learning. Campos *et al.* (1982), in their work with infants for whom the onset of independent mobility was inadvertently delayed, confirmed that some aspects of spatial, perceptual and cognitive development appear to be dependent on active, self-initiated exploration.

Motor actions may often obscure rather than hinder cognitive development and should not be taken as indices of underlying understanding or intelligence. It can, however, be argued that it is equally unwise to dismiss altogether the influence of motor actions in the child's cognitive development. Increasingly within the developmental literature, there are illustrations of the integrated nature of development and of interactions among the domains and pathways of development. Where for example a child has little or no independent mobility, it may not be just spatial knowledge which is impaired. Semantic development is related to some extent to experience, especially of verb forms, and the child may also show deficiencies in his movement vocabulary linked to his absence of movement experiences (Robinson and Feiber, 1988). To the extent that motor skills can be viewed as a learning pathway, their absence or dysfunction must be seen as having implications for the child's learning and for planning intervention.

12.2   Assessment of cognitive functioning

12.2.1   PLANNING THE ASSESSMENT

Children with cerebral palsy are a group for whom an assessment of cognitive functioning is often requested. This is because not only are they at risk of having some cognitive deficit, but their motor disabilities obscure their underlying cognitive abilities. Cognitive assessment may at certain stages in the child's development provide information which will help in parental adjustment and influence planning and decision making. It may also be seen as an ongoing process influencing and evaluating intervention and education programmes. Before embarking on an assessment of the child's cognitive abilities the following factors should be considered.

(a)   Purpose of assessment

As with any assessment it is important to be clear about the goals, as these will influence process, planning and product. For the child with cerebral palsy it may be important to differentiate essentially diagnostic and predictive questions, e.g. 'Is my child mentally handicapped?', 'Will she go to mainstream school/university?', from more descriptive/ prescriptive objectives concerned with elucidating the child's cognitive strengths and difficulties and selecting and evaluating strategies for enhancing her cognitive development.

(b)   The child's motor competences.

This may seem obvious in that a child's ability to act on her environment and in particular her ability to manipulate materials will affect her ability on most assessments, whether they employ formal psychometric tests, structured play strategies or more naturalistic observation. Correct positioning and appropriate seating (Chapter 10) are important not only for children with very severe motor disabilities who rely on these to achieve any manipulative skills, but also for children with milder disabilities, e.g. hemiplegia or diplegia, whose optimal performance on fine motor tasks may be dependent on stable seating. It is also important to be aware of the effort required by a child in achieving motor based activities. For example, it is easy for a 15-month-old child to build towers and 'post' shapes. She will do this casually in play without seeking or requiring external reward. The child with a movement difficulty, however, may achieve these skills but only with intense effort and concentration. She will not practise them in play and may not demonstrate her ability in an assessment situation if she is not sufficiently motivated. While such a child may appear to have adequate motor skills, her achievements on these tasks should not be compared directly with those of non-disabled peers, but should be considered within the context of the child's motor disabilities and motivational systems.

Speed and fluency of responses are also often used as indicators of underlying cognitive competence, e.g. a child who completes a puzzle more quickly than another is seen as being more cognitively competent in this respect. In children with cerebral palsy, as in non-disabled children, speed of response is related to cognitive abilities; however, any motor difficulties will also influence speed of response and cloud the issue significantly. Caution should be exercised in the use and interpretation of timed assessments in children with cerebral palsy.

(c)   The child's communicative competence

Where a child has difficulties in manipulating materials, the verbal communication channel may often be of particular importance in giving a window to the child's intellectual abilities. Individuals with more severe motor disabilities are, however, also likely to have some difficulties in communication. These may range from disorders that make speech mildly unintelligible, particularly to the assessor unfamiliar with the child, to those that require the child to use alternative communication systems (Chapter 13).

As with motor skills, the responses of a child who has difficulties in spoken language cannot be considered directly comparable to those of children with fluent communication skills. The additional effort in producing speech with dysarthria, or the complexities of using an alternative system, will influence length, fluency, content and complexity of verbal responses.

(d)   The child's sensory status

Knowledge of visual and auditory capacities is an essential prerequisite of any assessment of cognition. Some children with cerebral palsy will have visual and auditory problems which will not only add to but will complicate their sensori-motor disabilities.

Together with a clear knowledge of the objectives of assessment, information regarding the child's sensory status and motor and communication competence, will be essential both in helping in planning the assessment and in providing a context in which the child's responses may be interpreted. For children with severe or complex disabilities, a multidisciplinary approach to assessment offers the best opportunity of obtaining a comprehensive view of the child and an integration of information across domains.

12.3   Approaches to assessment

12.3.1   PSYCHOMETRIC TESTS

These are particularly likely to be used when the objectives of the assessment require a comparison of the child's functioning with her peer group and where some prediction of future functioning or of functioning in other settings is required. There are many drawbacks to the use of such tests with children with cerebral palsy. There is an assumption of sensory intactness and a reliance on motor responses, particularly in infant and early childhood tests. Timed responses are also commonly included in standardized cognitive assessments. The use of conventional scales is also limited by the lack of generalization of normative instruments to populations not included in the standardization sample. Most tests of standardization specifically exclude children with disabilities and yet some, e.g. Griffiths Scales (Griffiths, 1954), have their most extensive use in clinical assessment of children with disabilities. There is also a tendency for tests to overestimate intellectual deficit (Hunt, 1976).

As discussed above, children with severe physical disabilities may well have experiential deficits. Robinson and Feiber (1988) consider that these deficits can be 'pervasive, cumulative and synergistic', and that the child's lack of equal opportunities for acculturation should be considered in the same way as if the child had grown up in a different culture.

Violation of the assumptions underlying the development and use of standardized tests will clearly seriously affect the tests' validity. Where children have cerebral palsy, and particularly where their difficulties are severe and complex, generalization and predictions from the use of such tests will be much weaker than usual. In particular, the use of psychometric assessment with infants, e.g. Bayley (1969) and Griffiths (1954), presents many drawbacks. These instruments place a high reliance on motor responses, and predictive validity even for 'normal' infants is very poor. The prediction of intellectual functioning in an infant with cerebral palsy is possible only if the child has severe and global retardation, which would be evident without the use of tests.

The way in which items are selected for inclusion in tests also limits their applicability in assessments where the major concern is a description of the child's cognitive abilities linked to intervention and educational programmes. Test items are typically easily elicited, scorable and stable, but are not necessarily crucial to the child's development. Gaussen (1984) contends that the process of assessment and remediation is restricted by focusing on aspects of developmental change which are more fixed and less open to intervention.

12.4 Criterion-referenced approaches

These include a wide range of tests, checklists and scales, which are not norm-referenced and tend to reflect underlying curriculum objectives. Hence they relate more directly to intervention and education programmes. Examples for infant assessment include infant checklists, e.g. Stycar sequences (Sheridan, 1973), PIP charts (Jeffree and McConkey, 1976), early intervention curriculum checklists, e.g. Portage, Shearer and Shearer (1976) and the scales based on Piagetian theory (Escalona and Corman, 1969; Uzgiris and Hunt, 1975). For school age children the use of criterion-referenced assessment will include all tests given at school to evaluate a child's progress within the curriculum. In addition, assessment of children who are having difficulties in literacy and numeracy will tend to involve criterion-referenced tests.

Some of the drawbacks inherent in the use of psychometric approaches will also be found in many of the above, if used in a standard unmodified form. For younger children there is often an emphasis on motor responses and a bias towards eliciting or observing key milestones in development rather than focusing on the underlying cognitive processes. In older children there tends to be a reliance on competence in verbal and writing skills in sampling underlying knowledge. Many children with cerebral palsy are thus disadvantaged.

The major strength of criterion-referenced approaches is in flexibility of administration. If the curriculum objectives are appropriate to the child then it is usually possible to adapt the checklist of testing procedure to find out whether these objectives have been attained. An example here would be in assessing reading competence in a child with poor oral communication skills. The child may not cope with reading aloud or with answering comprehension questions, but given a multiple choice format could demonstrate word recognition skills and comprehension. The Piagetian frameworks also lend themselves well to adaptation, so while in initial design many tasks in the Uzgiris and Hunt (1975) assessment schedule are heavily reliant on skilled motor responses, considerable adaptation of both eliciting situation and response mode can allow for assessment of children with severe motor disabilities (Robinson and Feiber, 1988).

12.5   Assessment of attentional responses

The traditional approaches outlined above can offer little to the assessment of the child whose disabilities are so severe and complex as to restrict both movement and intentional communication. On a day-to-day basis, however, a child's alertness, persistence and selectivity of attention, goal directedness and social responses give both parents and professionals clues as to her underlying cognitions. Relatively recently there have been developments in the assessment of children with complex handicaps which use the child's orienting and attentional responses to stimuli to discern underlying cognitions. This is based on the work of developmental psychologists in investigating the cognitive competences of very young babies (Berg and Berg, 1979; Caron *et al.*, 1983). Initially this involved the use of psychophysiological measures. Both galvanic skin response changes and heart rate decelerations can provide an indication of attention to stimulation in infants and in older children and adults (Lewis *et al.*, 1966). Heart rate is the more reliable measure but is still subject to many other fluctuations in the child's state. It is perhaps best used in combination with observations of behavioural changes (Porges, 1979). Zelazo (1979) has further developed the use of the attention paradigm in clinical applications. Zelazo's procedure involves seating the infant on mother's knee in front of a small puppet theatre. An accurately timed sequence of stimuli is then presented and repeated. As the child develops an expectancy and habituates to the sequence, changes are introduced. Observers note a cluster of attentional and social responses and the procedure has been shown to be successful at detecting good perceptio-cognitive processing abilities in children whose overt competence appeared severely limited on more conventional measures (Kearsley, 1979; Zelazo, 1982).

Such approaches are of value only for a few children. They are time-consuming and require considerable resources either in terms of technology or in skilled observers. Gaussen and Stratton (1985) suggest that such assessment techniques should be made available in specialist centres. They are, however, less likely to be a part of everyday assessment in an intervention programme.

12.6 The use of microtechnology

Microtechnology provides an extension of attempts to make use of a child's limited response repertoire in assessment. It allows maximum use to be made of minimum responses. Any reliable voluntary action which the child can produce can be used to access touch screens, single or multiple switches or joysticks, to operate a microcomputer. Given appropriate software there can be a carefully graded presentation of stimuli and with the use of scanning or sequential presentation, the child can demonstrate knowledge of a range of concepts. There is a software package available for use with preschool children with special needs (Douglas, 1990). For older children microtechnology will enable them to cope with a range of multiple choice items and more sophisticated children can use alphabetic and number systems to access the computer.

The use of microtechnology in assessment does require that work has been done to enable the child to use a switch and cope competently with the strategies used, e.g. directional push of a joystick, multiple switch use, waiting for a scanning arrow, waiting for stimulus changes (see also Chapter 14). This approach to assessment will therefore be most useful when microcomputer use is part of the child's everyday learning programme.

12.7   Parental roles in assessment

It is increasingly appreciated that cognitive competence is not simply a characteristic of an infant, but develops in a social setting in interactions with carers (Brinker and Lewis, 1982). The limited response repertoire of an infant with a disability (Brooks-Gunn and Lewis, 1982), together with parents' attitudes and feelings (Bell, 1980), may result in significant disruption of the parent–infant interactions system for an infant with cerebral palsy. It is therefore essential that assessment of early cognitive functioning takes place within this system. The infant's key carer (usually mother) should not merely be present during the assessment, but be actively involved in engaging the infant in social and toy play. Not only does this relationship provide an essential context for both elicitation and interpretation of information regarding the infant's cognitive abilities, but it should provide the focus for intervention in early infancy.

Older children's competence and autonomy in play will also be influenced by their parental relationships and the presence or absence of a parent. Where a child has severe motor or communication difficulties, she may have greater and more persistent emotional and practical dependence on her parent for support and for facilitation and interpretation of responses.

Parents also have an intimate knowledge of their child based on observations and interactions on a daily basis over the child's life. It is the assessor's role to provide a framework and ask questions in a way which enables parents to share their knowledge. Parents must also be seen as having a primary interest in the assessment. Their needs to develop a better understanding of their child can sometimes best be met via a partnership approach to assessment. Here parent and professional plan, carry out and evaluate assessment together, usually over a period of time. While such approaches would not be welcomed by all parents, they are particularly appropriate where linked to intervention programmes which involve a parent–professional partnership.

As the child matures, parents continue to have a keen interest in all aspects of her education and in assessments. Other workers, e.g. teachers, will, however, take on some of the earlier parenting roles in providing information and support for the child and in working in partnership.

12.8 Child-referenced assessment

As outlined above, the assessment of children with severe motor difficulties will usually require significant modification and individualization of approach. While standard measures may provide the starting point or basis for these assessments, the focus inevitably changes from a comparison of the child's performance with that of others (norm-referenced) or with the test itself (criterion-referenced), to the performance of the child herself across time and settings. Child-referenced assessments have been advocated and developed for use with infants with special needs (Dubose *et al.*, 1977; Brinker and Lewis, 1982; Robinson and Fieber, 1988).

Essentially, a child-referenced approach to assessment involves the assessor in a continuing interaction with the child or parent–infant dyad. The assessor acts by setting and testing hypotheses and continually modifying strategies according to the child's responses. The focus is not simply on the child's response to a standard stimulus but includes a description of her problem solving strategies and a characterization of the range of her abilities. In a child-referenced assessment the process is given as much if not more weight than the product. These approaches are, therefore, particularly valuable in enabling those involved closely with a child, e.g. parents or teachers, to gain insights into the child's learning processes. Child-referenced approaches can link very directly into intervention programmes and can provide information not only about the child's cognitive status but also about her needs for environmentally based learning opportunities.

The use of child-referenced techniques makes much higher demands on the knowledge and skill of the assessor than the use of standard assessment formats. The assessor must have a working knowledge of child cognitive development and an awareness of the theoretical notions underpinning any standard assessment which form the basis of the assessment. Without this any modifications made may substantially alter the content validity of the assessment. It is also essential for those involved in assessment to understand the potential relationships between the child's disabilities and the development of her cognitive abilities. Sensory and motor disabilities such as those present in children with cerebral palsy can significantly affect learning experiences and opportunities. Different pathways may be taken in concept development. An example can be found in early number skills where non-handicapped children's performance in counting has been found to have been facilitated by opportunities to touch materials (Gelman, 1980). A child with manipulation difficulties will often be expected to use vision only in counting. It is important that the assessor is aware that visual counting is a more difficult task and that the child is taking a different pathway towards developing her early number concept.

It is also essential during an assessment of a child with a complex motor disability to incorporate a clear understanding of how the child's disabilities affect her responses and how modifications in response expectation or positioning may be helpful. It is not only motor factors which must be taken into consideration but also motivational factors. The child who finds movement difficult may fail at a task not because of motor incompetence but because of insufficient motivation.

During the process of a child-referenced assessment, modifications may be made to the stimuli presented, the response required or to the procedures adopted. Modifications in stimuli are usually made to enable the child to perceive or manipulate them more effectively. Materials may be made larger or lighter. For example, a baby may be able to lift a lighter rattle to the mouth or a bead on the end of a string may improve grasp for string pulling. Scanning or pointing may be facilitated by cutting up a page of pictures and rearranging them within the child's reach and visual range.

Modification of the responses required of the child involves the assessor in making use of the child's repertoire and potential repertoire of responses in a way which is appropriate to the task in question. Eye pointing may be used in children with severe motor difficulties that restrict their upper limb movement and verbal communication. At an early level eye gaze can be used as an indicator of interest and attention. In investigating object permanence, for example, the assessor may use persistence of visual interest as one indicator that the child is aware of a favoured object's presence under a cloth. At a more sophisticated level eye pointing must become specific and intentional. This is a skill a child needs to learn and it may be necessary to teach this prior to its use in assessment. Movement approximations may also be employed where children have motor difficulties. This relies on an assessor being able to interpret the intent of the child's movement even if the task goal was not achieved. Assisted movement provides an extension of this. The assessor gives minimal and partial assistance according to the child's intended movement. For children with no movement it is still possible to use guided movement based on the child's verbal, non-verbal or pre-verbal communication. These approaches are valuable, not only in assessment, but also as part of intervention where the child's sensory experiences in learning are enhanced.

Affective responses may also be taken as indicators of understanding in children with limited response repertoires. Surprise at violation of an expectancy or a smile at a funny picture may all give clues to underlying understanding. Children with cerebral palsy may, however, have atypical facial expression and limited control over smiles, which may overflow into jaw thrust. For many children a major aspect of the cognitive assessment-intervention programme will involve establishing clear readable responses, and much teaching and learning will be essential for both child and assessor. The rate at which children learn will, of course, be a valuable indicator as to underlying cognitive ability.

Procedural modifications are commonly employed in administering standard tests to children with disabilities. They may involve administering only a part of the test, for example, the use of only the verbal scale of the Wisc with children with motor disabilities or alterations in time constraints within the tests, or changes in seating and positioning. The use of additional reinforcers to enhance the child's motivation is a procedural modification which may also be employed in assessment of children with disabilities.

Child-referenced assessments are complex and time-consuming. They demand considerable expertise of the assessor. They are, however, capable of providing information which facilitates an understanding of the child's cognitive processes and is directly useful in intervention. While in children with severe motor difficulties there are major restrictions in the use of any assessment for comparison with non-disabled peers or for prediction of future functioning, a good quality child-referenced assessment can provide information which is helpful in parent counselling and in planning for placements. The major value of assessment is, however, in providing a description of the child's cognitive functioning which can be used, not just in educational intervention, but also in therapy programmes designed to enhance the child's physical and communication skills.

13 *Communication*

13.1 Assessment

Assessment should give a thorough idea of the child's development of language and communication, his rate of learning and, if alternative communication systems are necessary, the most efficient ways for the child to access those systems. Jones *et al.* (1990) point out that in addition to a developmental assessment, children with physical handicap should also be assessed in terms of the severity of the disability and how this affects functioning.

13.1.1 SOCIAL INTERACTION

The assessment of social interaction provides a framework for the assessment of other aspects of communication. Whatever the age of the child to be assessed, his motivation to communicate and his level of non-verbal skills give valuable information as to the potential level of sophistication which he can be expected to reach. A child's social interaction must be assessed in social situations so that his interpersonal relationships and the type and quality of communication that he elicits from others can be considered. The assessment should be functional and should be conducted in partnership with the child's parents, so that they themselves can become more aware of the child's social strategies and use these as a base-line to help him move forward.

It is important to note the strategies the child uses to initiate, respond to and maintain social interaction. Does he use eye contact, vocalization, body movements, extension and so on, language, or a combination of these? Is the child able to take part in turn-taking activities, and if so, does his timing enable him to participate fully or does slowness of response cause the interaction to break down? Is the child able to hold his attention on the salient speaker or feature in the environment, and is he able to make others in his environment aware of his interest and attention by gaze, direction and body posture? While assessing social interaction, it is important to help the child to control his position so that his body movements in response do not, as far as possible, end in uncontrolled movements. It may be advisable to assess social interaction in a variety of positions so that people in the child's environment are aware of the most favourable position for interacting. Even when a child's most efficient position has been found, his range of movements will still be restricted, and it is important to watch carefully for minute changes in facial expression, eye position and so on.

(a)   Intentionality

Most parents will know when their child is hungry or happy, or requiring attention. Discussing with the parents the strategies the child uses to convey these, whether intentional or pre-intentional, is useful for two reasons. Firstly, it gives the information needed for a base-line of communicative behaviour that the parents can use to help them recognize intentional behaviours and reinforce pre-intentional behaviours, so that they become intentional. Secondly, it may heighten the parents' awareness of minute changes in the child's behaviour and may also heighten their confidence in their ability to understand their child.

13.1.2.   LANGUAGE

It is important to assess language in a way that will be useful to the person with cerebral palsy. Standard scores and age levels may have their uses, but functional assessment will give guidelines for helping the person with cerebral palsy to maximize his communication. During assessment it is important that the child knows what is expected of him. Attention and consistent responses must be established.

(a)   Symbolism

The child is able to show evidence of his representational thought from the age of about 7 months, when object permanence begins to emerge. Subsequently the child not only remembers the functions of everyday objects, he is able to demonstrate these, e.g. he drinks out of a cup, pretends to brush his hair with a brush, and from about 15 months of age he is able to use these everyday objects in simple pretend play, for example brushing a doll's hair. Also at around this age level the child will begin to appreciate pictures and indicate his recognition that they represent objects in his environment. It is at roughly this level of symbolism that the child becomes able to recognize auditory signals as representing objects and features of his environment. This progression from the very concrete to the more abstract representational level is crucial to the development of language, which is a highly abstract and arbitrary symbol system. The child with cerebral palsy may not have had the opportunity to play in a representative way due to his physical difficulties, and during assessment it will be necessary to facilitate the child's demonstration of the level of symbolism that he has reached. It may be necessary to use eye pointing and/or a yes/no response to hidden objects and doll play to establish the child's representational level.

(b)   Comprehension

In order to assess the understanding of language, a consistent, reliable response, a basic yes/no, or on/off, at least is required. According to the child's age level and language level, most assessment methods can be adapted to provide information about comprehension of vocabulary, sentence length and grammatical complexity. For example, a common test format is for the child to pick one picture out of three or four. BPVT (British Picture Vocabulary Test), TROG (Test of Reception of Grammar) and CARROW pictures can be numbered 1 to 4 so that the child can indicate the number on a board or computer, he can eye point to the pictures cut up and stuck on an Etran frame, or he can use an on/off switch to indicate yes or no, as the tester points to each picture. For younger children, less formal assessments such as the Derbyshire Language Scheme can be adapted for eye pointing, e.g. I am going to put baby on the bed – show me baby and bed. At all times it is necessary to be aware of positioning and optimizing the child's movement and responses, particularly where test results are negative it is important to check working practices. Where it is not possible to obtain a consisitent, reliable response, it is important to inform others that this has not been possible, and that a reliable assessment has not taken place, rather than to suggest that the child's language levels are low.

(c)   Expressive language

In a child using vocal language, the range of vocabulary and average sentence length, grammatical complexity and patterns of use can be assessed with relative ease, using the usual range of tests and linguistic analysis of a data base. For the non-vocal child, or a child using both vocal and non-vocal means of communication, formal testing may be inadequate. For a full assessment the following are required.

1. List of vocabulary used, then test outside that range to see if the child can innovate.
2. List of types of sentence structure or signal combinations in the case of augmentative communication.

3. List of strategies, e.g. using a 'not' picture to signify opposite to etc.
4. List of the functions for which language is used, e.g. regulating the environment, contact, etc. (Halliday, 1975).

(d) Speech

In assessing the oral movements and linguistic systems required for speech, feeding history and current feeding behaviour should be taken into consideration. (This is more fully described in Chapter 11.) Speech difficulties in a child with cerebral palsy may be due to dysarthria which, if moderate to severe, may preclude the development of adequate oral communication. If mild, intelligibility may be affected by slurring or sluggishness of mouth movement, but in this case speech therapy may help to increase intelligibility. The following areas should be assessed.

1. Breath control – the number of words or syllables that the child can produce on one breath, and whether the breath breaks occur at relevant semantic boundaries.
2. Volume – is volume adequate for intelligibility and can a range of volume be achieved? Does appropriate volume diminish towards the end of sentences or after a period of discourse?
3. Pitch – is there sufficient control over the modulation of pitch to produce a variety of intonation patterns?
4. Speed and time – is the overall speed of delivery of speech correct, not too fast and not too slow? Is the child able to make timely responses to the conversation directed to him?
5. Production of speech sounds – is the child able to produce the full range of speech sounds accurately? Does accuracy diminish towards the end of a breath, a sentence, or a period of discourse?

It is important to assess whether the above factors change according to tiredness, illness, etc.

(e) Phonology

Children with cerebral palsy are as prone as children without physical disability to developmental problems in their sound system. As he learns language, the child acquires a set of rules by which words are represented by sound – this is the phonology system. Problems in the development of this system may be developmental or secondary to poor auditory attention, as a result of poor mobility. An assessment is carried out by analysing a sample of the child's connected speech in terms of linguistic rules and processes.

13.2   Praxis

It is possible that a child may, in addition to his other physical difficulties, experience problems in motor organization and planning for oral movements. The fine sequenced movements required for oral communication may be severely affected by this difficulty.

The presence of dyspraxia is assumed if, while being able to make the full range of mouth movements spontaneously when the movements are 'automatic', the child is unable to organize movements voluntarily. For example, the child may be able to laugh, chew, etc., but when asked to smile or to move his jaw round and round, is unable to produce the correct response in the absence of any difficulty in understanding the task. The assessor should establish the child's ability to make mouth movements by observation of the child in a spontaneous situation, e.g. mealtimes, play, etc., and then subsequently ask the child to reproduce mouth movements in imitation or following description. It is usual for dyspraxia to be suspected if the child is unable to achieve this target in imitation, if he appears to be 'groping' for the appropriate mouth movement, or if his responses are patchy and inconsistent.

Dyspraxia is usually defined as being an impairment of organization of movement in the absence of physical impairment. However, it is possible for dyspraxia to overlay the neurological problem and affect the child's ability to acquire the full range of speech sounds. Dyspraxia also affects the speed at which the child is able to modify his speech, which may mean that prolonged periods of speech therapy are required. If the presence of dyspraxia is established, the therapist needs to assess the range of sounds the child is able to produce currently, and whether those sounds deteriorate in connected speech.

13.2.1   COMMUNICATION STRATEGIES

If it is considered that a child would benefit from a communication aid, a complex and detailed assessment must take place. Jones *et al.* (1990) provide a detailed model of such an assessment, which takes account of mobility, posture, accessing skills, vision and eye movements, hearing, symbolic and verbal comprehension and communicative modes and functions. They emphasize that, in addition, the child's environment should be viewed for its potential for adapting to a communication system.

In addition to the skills mentioned above, it is also important to assess attention and motivation to communicate. The child for whom learning to communicate is fraught with difficulties will need to use his attention optimally. Eye pointing, for example, requires a high degree of dyadic or triadic attention, which switches from person to board and back to person and so on. Cooper *et al.* (1978) provide a detailed developemental sequence of attention skills.

The child who has been accustomed to using a passive/non-passive method of communication such as silent/cry, still/smile to indicate pleasure and displeasure may take some time to begin to be motivated to convey other, more specific, ideas, especially if doing so involves much greater effort. Therefore, the assessor must note the child's current method of communication and whether it may help or hinder more sophisticated communication skills.

13.3   Principles of communication facilitation

Communication occurs all day and every day, and the facilitation of communication in children with cerebral palsy should reflect this by recognizing that the family and teachers are the child's best resource. Regular sessions of speech therapy which do not include the child's significant others may lead the parents to feel that only the therapist can work on communication. This would, perhaps, discourage the amount of time spent in communication with the child. Written programmes may cause stress; they have to be read and assimilated into the parents' child-rearing practices. The programme writer's style of interaction with children may not correspond with that of the parents. If they attempt to adhere to the programme, their interaction may become stilted and unnatural, or they may abandon the programme, feel guilt, and their relationship with the child and therapist may suffer as a result. The best therapy takes place in a 'triple alliance' with information flowing freely in all directions.

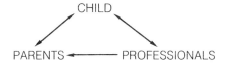

As experts on their child, the parents can be equal partners in the facilitation process with the therapist, who is the expert in the field of communication development in general. Following the initial assessment period, in which all parties join, the 'team' can make joint decisions about appropriate strategies for improving communication. These decisions can then be written down as an *'aide-mémoire'* as distinct from a 'programme'.

13.3.1   SOCIAL INTERACTION

The foundations of socialization are laid down in the first year, but the child continues to learn social rules until adulthood. Not all people master these rules completely.

Prescriptive therapy ideas may disturb the delicate balance of the social relationship between the child and his significant others. It is preferable to discuss with the parents the range of activities that would help the child move on to the next stage of development, and then assist them in their decisions about which activities to use and in which way.

Children with cerebral palsy may need facilitation in the following behaviours.

(a)   Intentional behaviour

Parents interpret children's behaviour as being meaningful until it becomes so. Poor physical ability may result in the range of behaviours the parents can interpret being limited. Also, if there is little obvious feedback from the child, the parent's interpreting behaviour may diminish. Facilitation therefore may involve increasing the parent's awareness of pre-intentional or intentional behaviour. By explaining its importance, it may be possible to increase the likelihood of interpretation and the length of time parents are willing to spend interacting with their child.

(b)   Joint attention

For communication to take place, the participants must be able to share a frame of reference. In the early stages of language development, babies and children establish reference by looking and/or pointing and/or sound making. They also develop the ability to recognize reference by watching eye direction or pointing. (At around 9 months the baby can look at an object, towards his mother, and back to the object to indicate interest.) For the child with minimal control over his gaze direction and body movements, timely interception of glances will be difficult and his own attempts to establish reference may be thwarted.

Awareness of where the child's interest is directed can be heightened in therapy and the child can be helped to direct his gaze more positively. Pointing with fist or finger in reception as well as expression can be encouraged.

(c) Turn taking

Turn taking is beginning to be established from the time a mother jiggles her baby when he stops suckling. The burst–pause pattern is the precursor of conversational and social patterns. First imposed by parents, the turn-taking pattern is rapidly taken up by the child, who becomes an initiator. Turn taking can take place through any medium – vocal, body, eye, mouth movements, etc.

(d) Anticipation

Early language is learned through verbal routines in familiar situations. The baby comes to anticipate and expect events to follow the 'build up', e.g. dinner arrives after clattering of plates, cooking smells and preparation of the table. In contexts like these, the child begins to expect certain language strings, e.g. 'dinner's ready', 'wash your hands', 'sit down', etc. Having learned this framework, he can begin to recognize word boundaries when other situations arise, e.g. bedtime – 'wash your face'. 'lie down' (Bruner, 1975).

Anticipation can be assisted by expectation games, e.g. 'round and round the garden', and by the repetition of action songs, dressing rituals, etc.

(e) Facilitation

In facilitating communication, the following should be considered:

1. position –
    optimal for looking, moving and responding;
2. parents/carers' awareness of
    eye direction
    pre-intentional behaviour
    play behaviours that could be used in turn taking
    child's need to interact;
3. child's control of
    people by sounds
    environment by play.

13.3.2 SYMBOLIC PLAY

Symbolic play, pretending to bath, feed, brush dolly and teddy, indicates that the child has reached the level of representing objects. The development of symbolic play co-occurs with language development, e.g. large doll play occurs at roughly the same age as phrase understanding, indicating the child's level of abstraction.

The child with cerebral palsy may have had little opportunity to play symbolically, and play where the child's symbolic intentions are indicated, e.g. by eye pointing, can be encouraged. For example the carer says 'Do you want to put baby in the bath or in the bed?' The child points to the bed. The carer puts the baby in the bed.

This type of play also provides the child with some control over his environment and exposes him to a rich variety of vocabulary and sentence structure.

13.3.3   LANGUAGE

In the context of social interaction of the first and second year the child has the opportunity for abstracting basic early language structures, but impaired mobility presents problems. It will be necessary to make conscious decisions about changes in the child's environment from day to day, so that he has the opportunity to experience variety in vocabulary and language structure.

Many parents intuitively provide the child, during daily activities, with language he can understand for the most part, with new elements introduced gradually. They base their language on their knowledge of the child's current vocabulary. The child, therefore, receives 'comprehensible input' in an environment where he is able to make most sense of new vocabulary. Where parents are not sure of their child's understanding, because of his poor ability to respond, the input may peter out or lack quality. The parents will need to find the most accurate and consistent measure of their child's comprehension by watching his minute responses, sometimes in contextually controlled situations. They will need help and support to do this as it exceeds instinctive behaviour and involves extra time.

Much of the child's language is learned actively through play and daily activities. The child learns not only the names of objects, but also actions, e.g. run, clap, eat, etc., positions, e.g. in, on, under, etc., and qualities, e.g. big, red, long, etc. In facilitating language it is important to include all types of words and resist the temptation to restrict language to labels.

The verb phrase, i.e. not just the action words but all those around it, e.g. 'He **would have been running**' is, perhaps, the most important in sentence structure both receptively and expressively. It carries tense, negative and interrogative markers, e.g.:

she is eating
she is not eating
she was eating
was she eating?
she wasn't eating, was she?

Again the child's language acquisition will be helped if he has experience of as many activities as possible, and these activities are discussed in terms of past, present and future, positive and negative, statement and interrogative. Pronouns also are an important aspect of vocabulary.

The child should be provided with a thorough and systematic opportunity to learn all aspects of language. In covering semantic and syntactic areas, the dynamic nature of language should be considered.

Understanding is an active process, usually learned in the context of expressive, physical interaction with the environment – talking, showing, looking, etc. The child with cerebral palsy needs not only linguistic input but also, from a very early age, the opportunity to experiment with and verify the input he gets by using expression. Early opportunities for expression have been discussed in section 2.3.5a and methods of expression will be discussed below. However, opportunity for expression cannot be stressed too highly.

The child needs:

1. a method of signalling others to listen/watch;
2. a method of output, e.g. choices: two objects held up for him to eye point or using body to indicate electronically, etc.;
3. people in his environment who can interpret his looks, points, synthesized voice, etc.

13.3.4   MEANS OF EXPRESSION

(a) Speech

Speech may be the main or augmented form of expressing language. The child should be monitored throughout his early years and, if necessary, receive help with eating, drinking and vocal play.

Intelligible speech, though desirable, may not be possible while the child is still young. The emotional maturity and concentration of children over about 5 years is necessary for the practice in production of sounds, the self-monitoring of speech performance and the motivation to produce intelligible speech against considerable odds.

(b) *Augmented/alternative systems*

Opinions about augmented/alternative systems for children with cerebral palsy fall into roughly two camps.

1. The child should be given a system as soon as possible so as not to fail in communication, and to learn that he can be an active participant.
2. The child should not be given an augmentive system until absolutely necessary, as it singles him out from others, and makes it less likely that he will learn normal interactional skills.

It may be appropriate at this point to discuss some of the disadvantages and the advantages of an alternative system of communication.

Disadvantages
1. It is not a natural method of communication; child, parents and carers will have to learn the system.
2. Each new vocabulary item will be learnt specifically, opportunities for casual learning will be missed.
3. The child loses control over the choice of vocabulary.
4. The rhythm and spontaneity of oral interaction are disrupted.
5. The range of people with whom the child can communicate may be limited.

Advantages
1. However limited the alternative system, it is not as limiting as depriving the child of a system at all.
2. It is essential in establishing and maintaining a child's motivation to communicate.
3. It minimizes frustration and failure avoidance.
4. Children needing long-term alternative systems will benefit from early brushes with technology.
5. It is important for the child to experience control in communication and have opportunities to initiate.
6. A high technology aid may enhance the child's reputation among his peers.

The approach adopted to each individual child should be discussed thoroughly with the parents, and a decision made jointly, all parties keeping the best interest of the child in mind.

Alternative systems cannot merely be supplied. The child and family must gradually learn to use the system and adapt to it together. The type of system used will depend on the following.

1. Symbolic ability: according to the child's symbolic ability, the alternative system may use objects, pictures, symbols, e.g. Bliss, Makaton, words, letters or icons. The child may graduate from one system to another as he grows and matures. No system is intrinsically superior to any other as long as it suits the child's needs. However, some systems, e.g. letters and icons, can be more flexible than others, and this should be considered.
2. Physical ability: physical ability will determine the child's method of use of the system:

    (a) pointing, with head, eye, or other parts of the body, head sticks, etc.;

    (b) switching, knocking sideways, pushing down, pushing up, lowering, tilting, using light pressure, lift off, stroke, press on by any part of the body, head, foot, elbow, etc. (See Chapter 14 on microtechnology.)

Pointing and switching can be used to scan boards or code, e.g. the child indicates the column on one axis and the row on another axis, and the receiver works out the relevant sign. Pointing sticks and switches can be made, or the more sophisticated ones can be bought commercially. It is important to remember that the child will probably have more than one communication system in his life according to his needs.

Teaching should be gradual. The level that can be reached will depend on the child's intellectual ability, e.g. understanding of cause and effect, and his opportunity to use his system in a receptive environment.

There should be adequate training for parents and carers. This is an excellent example of the need for the therapist to work with the child through the parents. The therapist can introduce the family to the child's system, but the use of it is developed between parent and child, as well as the significant others. The child's extended family, friends, teachers, etc. should be included in learning how to understand the child's communication system.

14   *Microtechnology*

Technological advances in recent years have had profound implications for the development and independence of people with physical disabilities. All areas of life can potentially be enhanced.

14.1   Microcomputers

Microcomputers have, almost simultaneously, become smaller and more sophisticated in recent years. The lap-top computer is now commonplace and, with appropriate software and switching, can give the person with cerebral palsy opportunities for control and development using word processors.

For the young child most software is available for larger computer systems, such as the BBC Master, which cannot be wheelchair-borne. Again, with appropriate switching, these systems provide the child with a level of independence in play which they could not otherwise achieve. While toy play can be frustrating if the child is not able to manipulate the toys successfully, the computer provides an immediate, often quite exciting, response to the touch of a switch. Programs involving scanning, or use of more than one switch, introduce choice in play and the child is allowed the luxury of playing alone for several minutes.

The computer can also be used as a teaching aid as it is highly motivating.

14.1.1   VISUAL ATTENTION AND VISUAL TRACKING

Bright pictures often with an additional sound stimulus draw the child's attention to the screen and changes to the picture encourage the child to maintain visual contact. Some programs have a target picture moving randomly over the screen for the child to follow. More specific directional tracking programs can be found involving vertical or horizontal left to right movements to simulate eye direction used in reading.

14.1.2 CAUSE AND EFFECT

Using a touch screen which responds to physical contact providing immediate visual feedback, the child can begin to develop cause and effect. Gradually the distance between the switch and the screen can be increased so that the child is able to associate the switch press with an effect on the screen.

14.1.3 SEQUENCED ACTIONS

Some software gives the opportunity to learn that only when certain conditions pertain will a switch press produce an effect. Some software teaches that one switch must be pressed before another, introducing concepts of sequences, contingency and so on. These concepts are necessary for the use of scanning or coding communication aids.

14.1.4 LANGUAGE

Computers again provide motivational material which may enhance the development of the understanding and use of language.

Some programs have speech synthesis, so theoretically it is possible for the child to interact with the machine. However, speech synthesis tends to be of a fairly poor quality that requires interpretation and also a computer program cannot react dynamically to a child's communication attempts.

Programs have been developed which specifically teach verbs or prepositions and these may be useful aids for the child with restricted movement.

14.1.5 CONCEPT DEVELOPMENT

The child with restricted movement is not able to develop ideas through play with puzzles, matching games, size grading toys, and so on. A wide range of software is available to teach number, shape, colour and letter concepts. The child is able to play alone and work at her own pace and most programs incorporate a visual and auditory reward at the end of the game. Some programs provide scores to enable parents or teachers to monitor progress.

14.1.6 PHYSICAL SKILL

Again, the motivational aspect of the computer can be used to teach and encourage physical development. A child may be encouraged to raise his head if doing so breaks a light beam and operates a switch which ensures a visual and auditory reward. Or the child may be encouraged to roll on to a switch for the same result.

Some switches will encourage directional movements of the hands, skills which can later be applied to the operation of a wheelchair.

14.2 Software

In Britain the decision to equip all schools with computers for children's use has resulted in a decade of growth in the development of software to cater for all types of needs. Some software houses will design material to fulfil specific requirements, but the bulk of the best work goes to the mainstream market. It is regrettable that graphics on programs aimed at the disabled population tend to be very poor when compared with 'arcade' type video games designed for home computers. It is to be hoped that this situation will improve in the future.

14.3 Switches

Using an interface, any switching device that has the appropriate plug can be used to activate programs. This provides versatility when using computers with different people or for one person's differing needs.

Switches are available which can be operated by any part of the body, including the tongue, eye movements, sucking and blowing actions, blinking or the voice. The part of the body which works the best may not always be the most ideal for switch operation, and the switch may need to be situated in a special position on the child's seating and other equipment. A bio-engineer is best equipped to assess maximum function.

While the computer fulfils a versatile and general function, some technology has a specific purpose.

14.3.1 COMMUNICATION AIDS

There is now a range of commerically made communication aids. They range from machines using short periods of recorded voice to machines which can produce long stretches of synthesized voice. Each has its own advantages and disadvantages for users and listeners and can be successfully used if the correct balance between them is found.

Some listeners find even good quality synthesized voice difficult, but it is this which can provide the most creative opportunities for the user.

Recorded voice which can be made appropriate to the user, e.g. a young female voice for a little girl, is limited in that the aid cannot generate language from the input, and the user is obliged to reiterate the pre-recorded phrases.

14.3.2 MOBILITY AIDS

Electronic controls for wheelchairs are available which require minimal movement to start, stop and change direction. They can give some experience of mobility and valuable independence.

14.3.3 ENVIRONMENTAL CONTROLS

These sophisticated devices can operate lights, curtains, alarms and switch electrical items on and off. The young adult may find a much needed degree of independence in her life through these controls, which will allow her to spend short periods of time alone without having close contact with helpers.

References

Abercrombie, M. C. J. (1964) *Perceptual and Visuo-Motor Disorders in Cerebral Palsy*, Spastics Society, Heinemann, London.

Aicardi, J. and Goutieres, F. (1972) Multicystic Encephalomalacia of Infants and Its Relation to Abnormal Gestation and Hydranencephaly. *Journal Neurological Science*, **15**, 357–73.

Aicardi, J. (1980) Seizures and Epilepsy In Children under Two Years of Age; in *The Treatment of Epilepsy* (ed J. Tyler), Lippincott, Philadelphia.

Aicardi, J. (1988) Clinical Approach to the Management of Intractable Epilepsy. *Developmental Medicine and Child Neurology*, **30**(4), 429–40.

Aicardi, J. (1990) Epilepsy in Brain Injured Children. *Developmental Medicine and Child Neurology*, **32**(3), 191–202.

Ainsworth, M. D. S. and Bell, S. M. (1974) Mother Infant Interaction and the Development of Competence, in *The Growth of Competence* (eds K. J. Connolly and J. S. Bruner), Academic Press, New York.

Alberman, E. D. (1963) Birthweight and Length of Gestation in Cerebral Palsy. *Developmental Medicine and Child Neurology*, **5**, 388–94.

Alston, J. and Hancock, J. (1986) The Effect of Pencil Barrel Shape and Pupil Barrel Preference on Hold or Grip in 8 Year Old Pupils. *British Journal of Occupational Therapy*, **49**, 242–4.

Alston, J. and Taylor, J. (1984) *The Handwriting File: Diagnosis and Remediation of Handwriting Difficulties*, Learning Development Aids, Wisbeck.

American Academy of Paediatrics (1982) Policy Statement: the Doman Delacato Treatment of Neurologically Handicapped Children. *Pediatrics*, **5**, 810–11.

Anastasiow, N. J. (1984) Handicapped Preschool Children: Peer Contacts, Relationships and Friendships, in *Friendships in Normal and Handicapped Children* (eds T. Field, J. Roopwarine and M. Segal), Ablex Publishing, Norwood, New Jersey.

Anderson, E. M. (1973) *The Disabled School Child*, Methuen, London.

Anderson, E. M. (1979) Helping SBH Pupils with Handwriting. Special Education Forward Trends. *British Journal of Special Education*, **6**(1).

Anderson, E. M., Clarke, I. and Spain, B. (1982) *Disability in Adolescence*, Methuen, London.

Armstrong, D. and Norman, M. G. (1974) Periventricular Leucomalacia in Neonates. Complications and Sequelae. *Archives of Disease in Childhood*, **49**, 367.

Baker, B. L. (1980) Training Parents as Teachers of Their Disabled Child, in *The Ecosystem of the Sick Child* (eds S. Salzinger, J. Antrobus and J. Slick),

Academic Press, New York.

Banker, B. Q. (1961) Cerebral Vascular Disease in Infancy and Childhood. *J. Neuropath. Exp. Neurol.*, **20**, 127–40.

Banker, B. and Larroche, J. C. (1962) Periventricular Leucomalacia of Infancy. *Arch. Neurol.*, **7**, 32.

Barsch, R. (1964) The Handicapped Ranking Scale among Parents of Handicapped Children. *American Journal of Public Health*, **54**, 1560–7.

Barsch, R. (1968) *The Parent of the Handicapped Child*, Thomas, Springfield, Illinois.

Bax, M. (1964) Terminology and Classification of Cerebral Palsy. *Developmental Medicine and Child Neurology*, **6**, 295.

Bax, M. and Oswin (1967) *The Handicapped Adolescent*. Paper read at St Christopher's Hospital for Children, Philadelphia.

Bax, M. (1990) Puzzles about Epilepsy. *Developmental Medicine and Child Neurology*, **32**(10), 847–8.

Bayley, N. (1969) *Bayley Scales of Infant Development*, Psychological Corporation, New York.

Beghi, E., Bollini, P., Di Mascio, R., Cerisola, N., Merloni, T. and Manghi, E. (1987) Effects of Rationalising Drug Treatment of Patients with Epilepsy and Mental Retardation. *Developmental Medicine and Child Neurology*, **29**(3), 363–70.

Bell, P. B. (1980) *Characteristics of Handicapped Infants: A Study of the Relationship between Child Characteristics and Stress as Reported by Mothers*. Unpublished doctoral dissertation, University of North Carolina, Chapel Hill, North Carolina.

Bell, C. and Quintal, J. (1985) A Life Skills Programme for Physically Disabled Adolescents. *Canadian Journal of Occupational Therapy*, **52**(5), 235–9.

Berg, W. K. and Berg, K. M. (1979) Psychophysiological Development in Infancy: State, Sensory Function and Attention, in *Handbook of Infant Development* (ed. J. D. Osofsky), John Wiley, New York.

Bertenthal, B. I. and Campos, J. J. (1987) New Directions in the Study of Early Experience. *Child Development*, **58**, 560–7.

Beveridge, B. and Brinker, R. (1980) An Ecological-Development Approach to Communication in Retarded Children, in *Language Disorders in Children* (ed. M. Jones), MTP Press, London.

Blacher, J. (1984) *Severely Handicapped Young Children and their Families*, Academic Press, London.

Blacher, J. and Meyers, C. E. (1983) A Review of Attachment Formation and Disorder of Handicapped Children. *American Journal of Mental Deficiency*, **87**(4), 359–71.

Bobath, B. (1963) Treatment Principles and Planning in Cerebral Palsy. *Physiotherapy*, **49**, 122.

Bobath, B. and Bobath, K. (1975) *Motor Development in Different Types of Cerebral Palsy*, Heinemann Medical Books Ltd, London.

Bobath, B. and Bobath, K. (1984) The Neurodevelopmental Treatment, in *Management of the Motor Disorders of Children* (ed. D. Scrutton). Spastics International Medical Publications, Philadelphia.

Bower, T. (1977) *The Perceptual World of the Child*, Fontana, London.

Bozynski, M. E., Nelson, M. N., Genaze, D., Rosati Skertich, C., Matalon, T., Vasan, U. and Naughton, P. (1988) Cranial Ultrasonography and the Prediction of Cerebral Palsy in Infants Weighing Less Than 1200 grams at Birth. *Developmental Medicine and Child Neurology*, **30**, 342–8.

Bradley, L. (1980) Reading, Spelling and Writing Problems, in *Helping Clumsy Children* (eds N. Gordon and I. McKinley), Churchill Livingstone, Edinburgh, pp. 135–44.

Brinker, R. and Lewis, M. (1982) Discovering the Competent Handicapped Infant. A Process Approach to Assessment and Intervention. *Topics in Early Childhood: Special Education*, **2**, 1–16.

British Association of Social Work (1985) *Housing and Social Work*.

Bromwich, R. M. (1976) Focus on Maternal Behaviour in Infant Intervention. *Journal of Orthopsychiatry*, **46**(3), 439–46.

Bromwich, R. (1981) *Working with Parents: An Interactional Approach*, Baltimore University Park Press.

Brooks-Gunn, J. and Lewis, M. (1982) Affective Exchanges Between Normal and Handicapped Infants and Their Mothers, in *Emotion and Interaction in High Risk Infants* (eds T. Field and A. Fogel), Erlbaum, Hillsdale, New Jersey.

Brown, C. (1954) *My Left Foot*, Secker & Warburg, London.

Brown, J. K. (1984) Disorders of the Central Nervous System, in *Textbook of Paediatrics*, 3rd edn (eds J. O. Forfar and G. C. Arneil), Churchill Livingstone, Edinburgh.

Brown, J. K., Purvis, R. J., Forfar, J. and Cockburn, F. (1974) Neurological Aspects of Perinatal Asphyxia. *Developmental Medicine and Child Neurology*, **16**, 567–80.

Bruner, J. S. (1966) *Towards a Theory of Instruction*, W. W. Norton, New York.

Bruner, J. S. (1972) The Nature and Uses of Immaturity. *American Psychologist*, 8 Aug.

Bruner, J. S. (1975) The Ontogenesis of Speech Acts. *Journal of Child Language*, **2**, 1–19.

Brunswic, M. (1984) Ergonomics of Seat Design. *Physiotherapy*, **70**, 40–3.

Campbell, D. D. (1973) Typewriting Contrasted with Handwriting: A Circumvention Study of Learning in Disabled Children. *J. Spec. Ed.*, 155–68.

Campos, J., Svejda, M., Campos, R. and Bertenthal, B. (1982) The Emergence of Self-produced Locomotion: Its Importance for Psychological Development in Infancy, in *Intervention with At Risk and Handicapped Infants. From Research to Application* (ed. D. Bricker), Baltimore University Park Press.

Caron, A. J., Caron, R. F. and Glass, P. (1983) Responsiveness to Relational Information as a Measure of Cognitive Functioning in Non-Suspect Infants, in *Infants Born at Risk: Physiological, Perceptual and Cognitive Processes* (eds T. Field and A. Sostek), Grune and Stratton, New York.

CERI/OECD (1987) *Handicapped Adult Status: Policy Issues and Practical Dilemmas*, Paris.

Clarke, R. (1974) Performing Without Competence. *Journal of Child Language*, **1**, 1.

Clarke, R. M. and Linnell, E. A. (1954) Prenatal Occlusion of the Internal Carotid Artery. *J. Neurology, Neurosurg. and Psych.*, **17**, 295 7.

Cocker, J., George, S. W. and Yates, P. O. (1965) Perinatal Occlusion of the Middle Cerebral Artery. *Developmental Medicine and Child Neurology*, **7**, 235–43.

Cooper, J., Moodley, M. and Reynell, J. (1978) *Helping Language Development*, Edward Arnold, London.

Corbett, J. and Pond, D. (1985) The Management of Epilepsy, in *Mental Handicap* (eds M. Craft, J. Bicknell and S. Hollins), Bailliere Tindall, London.

Cottam, P. and Sutton, A. (1986) *Conductive Education – A System for Overcoming Motor Disorder*, Croom Helm, London.

Crothers, B. and Paine, R. S. (1959) *The Natural History of Cerebral Palsy*, Harvard University Press, Cambridge, Mass.

Cruikshank, W. M. (1976) *Cerebral Palsy: A Developmental Disability*, Syracuse University Press, New York.

Cruikshank, W. M., Hallahan, D. and Bice, H. (1976) The Evaluation of Intelligence, in *Cerebral Palsy: A Developmental Disability*, (ed. W. M. Cruikshank), Syracuse University Press, New York.

Cunningham, C. and Davis, H. (1985) Early Parent Counselling, in *Mental Handicap* (eds M. Craft, J. Bicknell and S. Hoskins), Baillière Tindall, London.

Darling, R. B. and Darling, J. (1982) *Children who are Different: Meeting the Challenges of Birth Defects in Society*, C. V. Mosby, St Louis.

Davies, P. A. and Tizard, J. P. M. (1975) Very Low Birth Weight and Subsequent Neurological Defect with Special Reference to Spastic Diplegia. *Developmental Medicine and Child Neurology*, **17**, 3–17.

Decarie, T. B. (1969) A Study of the Mental and Educational Development of the Thalidomide Child, in *Determinants of Infant Behaviour, IV* (ed. B. Foss), Methuen, London.

deVries, J., Visser, G. and Prechtl, H. (1984) Fetal Motility in the First Half of Pregnancy, in *Continuity of Neural Functions from Prenatal to Postnatal Life* (ed H. F. R. Prechtl). Spastics International Medical Publications, Blackwell Scientific Publications Ltd., Oxford.

Doman, R. J., Spitz E. B., Zucman, E. *et al.* (1960) Children with Severe Brain Injuries, Results of Treatment. *J. Am. Med. Ass*, **174**(2), 257–62.

Donaldson, M. (1978) *Children's Minds*, Fontana, London.

Dubose, R., Langley, M. and Stagg, V. (1977) Assessing Severely Handicapped Children. *Focus on Exceptional Children*, **9**, 1–13.

Douglas, J. (1990) *Special Needs Assessment Software*, NFER Nelson, Windsor.

Eagle, R. S. (1985) Deprivation of Early Sensori-motor Experience and Cognition in the Severely Involved Cerebral Palsied Child. *Journal of Autism and Developmental Disorders*, **15**, 3.

Edwards, A. D., Reynolds, E. O. R., Richardson, C. E. and Wyatt, J. S. (1989) Estimation of Blood Flow Using Near Infrared Spectroscopy. *J. Physiol.*, **410**, 50.

Eibl-Eibesfeldt, I. (1970) *The Biology of Behaviour*, Holt, Reinhart & Wilson, New York.

Eimas, B. D. (1974) Linguistic Processing of Speech by Young Infants, in

Language Perspectives, Acquisition, Retardation and Intervention (eds R. L. Schiefelbusch and L. Lloyd), University Park Press, Baltimore.

Escalona, S.K. and Corman, H. (1969) *Albert Einstein Scales of Sensory-motor Development*. Albert Einstein College of Medicine of Yeshiva University, New York.

Evans, P. and Alberman, E. (1985) Recording the Motor Deficits in Cerebral Palsy. *Developmental Medicine and Child Neurology*, **27**, 404–6.

Fantz, R. L. (1966) Pattern Discrimination and Selective Attention as Determinants of Perceptual Development from Birth, in *Perceptual Development in Children* (eds A. J. Kidd and J. Rivoire), International Universities Press, New York.

Farber, B. (1975) Family Adaptations to Severely Mentally Retarded Children, in *The Mentally Retarded and Society: A Social Science Perspective* (eds J. Begab and S. A. Richardson), University Park Press, Baltimore.

Ferrer, I. and Navarro, C. (1978) Multicystic Encephalomalacia of Infancy. *J. Neurol. Sci.*, **38**, 179–89.

Field T., Roseman S., Destafano I., and Koewler J. H. (1981) Play Behaviours of Handicapped Preschool Children in the Prescence and Absence of Non-Handicapped Peers. *Journal of Applied Developmental Psychology*. **2**, 49–58.

Finnie, N. R. (1974) *Handling the Young Cerebral Palsied Child at Home*. Heinemann Medical Books, London.

Foley, H. (1990) The Treatment of Epilepsy in People with Multiple Handicap. *Archives of Disease in Childhood*, **65**, 453–7.

Forfar, J. O. and Arneil, G. C. (1984) *Textbook of Paediatrics*, 3rd edn, pp. 1666–70, Churchill Livingstone, Edinburgh.

Freeman, R. D. (1970) Psychiatric Problems in Adolescents with Cerebral Palsy. *Developmental and Medicine and Child Neurology*, **12**(1), 64–70.

Gaussen, T. (1984) Developmental Milestones or Conceptual Millstones: Some Practical and Theoretical Limitations in Infant Assessment Procedures. *Child Care Health and Development*, **10**, 99–115.

Gaussen, T. and Stratton, P. (1985) Beyond the Milestone Model: A Systems Framework for Infant Assessment. *Child Care Health and Development*, **11**, 131–50.

Gastaut, H. (1981) Proposal for the Revised Clinical and Electroencephalographic Classification of Epileptic Seizures. *Epilepsia*, **22**, 489–501.

Gelman, R. (1980) What Young Children Know about Numbers. *Educational Psychologist*, **15**, 54–68.

Gottman, J., Gonso, J. and Rasmussen, B. (1975) Social Interaction, Social Competence and Friendship in Children. *Child Development*, **45**(3), 709–18.

Greengross, W. (1980) *Sex and the Handicapped Child*, National Marriage Guidance Council, Rugby, UK.

Griffiths, R. (1954) *The Abilities of Babies*, University of London Press, London.

Guralnick, M. J. (1981) Programmatic Factors affecting Child–Child Social Interactions in Mainstreamed Preschool Programs. *Exceptional Education Quarterly*, **1**(4), 71–91.

Gustavson, K., Hagberg, B. and Sanner, G. (1969) Identical Syndromes of Cerebral Palsy in the Same Family. *Act. Paed. Scan.*, **58**, 330–40.

Hagberg, B., Hagberg, G. and Olow, I. (1975) The Changing Panorama of Cerebral Palsy in Sweden. *Acta Paediatrica Scand.*, **61**, 187–200.

Hagberg, B. and Hagberg, G. (1984) Prenatal and Perinatal Risk Factors in a Survey of 681 Swedish Cases, in *The Epidemiology of the Cerebral Palsies. Clinics in Developmental medicine. No. 87* (eds F. Stanley and E. Alberman), Blackwell, Oxford.

Hall, J. G. (1964) The Cochlea and Cochlear Nuclei in Neonatal Asphyxia. *Acta Otolaryngolica (Suppl.)*, **194**, 1–93.

Halliday, M. A. K. (1975) *Learning to Mean: Explorations in the Development of Language*, Edward Arnold, London.

Harrison, A. (1988) Spastic Cerebral Palsy; Possible Spinal Interneuronal Contributions. *Developmental Medicine and Child Neurology*, **30**, 769–80.

Hartup, W. W. (1974) Aggression in Childhood: Developmental Perspectives. *American Psychologist*, **29**(5), 336–41.

Hartup, W. W. (1978) Peer Interaction and the Process of Socialisation, in *Early Intervention and the Integration of Handicapped and Non-Handicapped Children* (ed. M. J. Guralnick), University Park Press, Baltimore.

Hartup, W.W. (1983) The Peer System, in *Handbook of Child Psychology Series* vol 4 (ed. P. Mussen), Wiley, New York.

Hegarty, S. (1982) Meeting Special Needs in the Ordinary School. *Education Research*, **24**(3), 174–81.

Hegarty, S., Pocklington, K. and Lucas, D. (1981) *Educating Pupils with Special Needs in the Ordinary School*, NFER Nelson, Windsor.

Henderson, S. (1961) *Cerebral Palsy in Childhood and Adolescence*. E and S Livingstone. Edinburgh and London.

HMSO (1986) *Disabled Persons (Services, Consultation and Representation) Act*, London.

Herndon, W., Troup, P., Yngve, M. and Sullivan, J. (1987) Effects of Neurodevelopmental Treatment on Movement Patterns in Children with Cerebral Palsy. *Journal of Pediatric Orthopedics*, **7**, 395–400.

Hewson, J. and Tizard, J. (1980) Parental Involvement and Reading Attainment. *British Journal of Educational Psychology*, **50**, 209–15.

Hirst, M. (1984) *Moving On: Transfer of Young People with Disabilities to Adult Services*, DHSS, 190, June.

Hirst, M. (1985) Social Security and Insecurity. Young People with Disabilities in the United Kingdom, *International Social Security Review March 1985*, Social Policy Research Unit, University of York, York.

Hirst, M. (1987) Careers of Young People with Disabilities between Ages 15 and 21 Years'. *Disability, Handicapped Society*, **2**, 1.

Holt, K. S. and Reynell, J. K. (1967) *Assessment of Cerebral Palsy Vol. 2*, Lloyd Luke, London.

Hodgeson, A., Clunies-Ross, L. and Hegarty, S. (1984) *Teaching Pupils with Special Educational Needs in the Ordinary School*, NFER Nelson, Windsor.

Hops, H. and Greenwood, C. R. (1981) Social Skill Deficits in (ed E. J. Mash and L. G. Terdal), *Behavioural Assessment of Childhood Disorders*, Guilford Press, New York.

Hunt, J. (1976) Environmental Risk in Foetal and Neonatal Life and Measured

Intelligence. In *Origins of Intelligence in Early Childhood* (ed. M. Lewis), John Wiley, New York.

Huttenlocher, P. (1976) Ketonemia and Seizures; Metabolic and Anticonvulsant Effects of Two Ketogenic Diets in Childhood Epilepsy. *Pediatric Research*, **10**, 536–40.

Ingram, T. T. S. (1964) *Paediatric Aspects of Cerebral Palsy*, E. and S. Livingstone, Edinburgh and London.

Jeavons, P. and Aspinall, A. (1985) *The Epilepsy Reference Book*. Harper and Row, London.

Jeffree, O. and McConkey, R. (1976) *PIP Developmental Charts*, Hodder and Stoughton, Sevenoaks, Kent.

Jesurum, C. A., Levin, G. S., Sullivan, W. R. and Stevens, D. (1980) Intracranial Haemorrhage In Utero and Thrombocytopenia. *J. Paediatrics*, **97**, 695–6.

Jones, O. H. (1980) Prelinguistic Communication Skills in Downs Syndrome and Normal Infants, in *High Risk Infants and Children, Adult and Peer Interactions* (eds T. Field, S. Goldberg, D. Stern and A. Sostek), Academic Press, New York.

Jones, N. J. (1983) An Integrative Approach to Special Educational Needs. *Forum*, **25**(2), 36–9.

Jones, S., Jolleff, N. and McConachie, H. (1990) A Model for Assessment of Children for Augmentative Communication Systems. *Child Language Teaching and Therapy*, **6**, 3.

Kagan, J. (1970) Attention and Psychological Change in the Young Child. *Science*, **170**, 826–32.

Kearsley, R. B. (1979) Iatrogenic Retardation: A Syndrome of Learned Incompetence, in *Infants at Risk: Assessment of Cognitive Functioning* (eds R. B. Kearsley and I. E. Sigel), Erlbaum, New Jersey.

Kent, A., Massie, B., Newman, B. and Tuckey, L. (1984) *Day Centres for Young Disabled People*, RADAR, London.

Killen, M. and Uzgino, I. C. (1981) Imitation of Actions with Objects. The Role of Social Meaning. *Journal of Genetic Psychology*, **138**(2), 219–29.

Kogan, K., Taylor, N. and Turner, P. (1974) The Process of Interpersonal Adaptation between Mothers and their Cerebral Palsied Children. *Developmental Medicine and Child Neurology*, **16**, 518–27.

Kopp, C. and Shaperman, J. (1973) Cognitive Development in the Absence of Object Manipulation during Infancy. *Developmental Psychology*, **9**, 430.

Laborde, P. R. and Seligman, M. (1983) Individual Counselling with Parents of Handicapped Children, in *The Family with a Handicapped Child* (ed. M. Seligman), Strune and Gratton, New York.

Lamb, M. E. (1983) Fathers of Exceptional Children, in *The Family with a Handicapped Child* (ed. M. Seligman), Strune and Gratton, New York.

Larroche, J. C. and Amiel, C. (1966) Thrombose de l'artère Sylvienne à la Période Néonatale. *Arch. Fr. Pédiat.*, **23**, 257–74.

Larroche, J. C. (1986) Fetal Encephalopathies of Circulatory Origin. *Biol. Neonate*, **50**, 61–74.

Levene, M., Wigglesworth, J. and Dubowitz, V. (1981) Cerebral Structure and

Intraventricular Haemorrhage in the Neonate; a Real-Time Ultrasound Study. *Archives of Disease in Childhood*, **56**, 416–24.

Levene, M., Wigglesworth, J. and Dubowitz, V. (1983) Haemorrhagic Periventricular Leucomalacia in the Neonate. A Real-Time Ultrasound Study. *Pediatrics*, **71**(5), 794–7.

Levene, M. I., Gands, C., Grindulis, H. and Moore, J. R. (1986) Comparison of Two Methods of Predicting Outcome in Perinatal Asphyxia. *Lancet*, **1**, 67–9.

Lewis, H., Kagan, J., Campbell, H. and Kalafat, J. (1966) The Cardiac Response as a Correlate of Attention in Infants. *Child Development*, **37**,63–71.

Lewis, V. (1987) *Development and Handicap*, Blackwell, Oxford.

Lindsay, J., Ounstead, C. and Richards, P. (1987) Hemispherectomy for Childhood Epilepsy; A 36-Year Study. *Developmental Medicine and Child Neurology*, **29**, 592–600.

Little, W. J. (1862, reprinted in 1958) On the Influence of Abnormal Parturition, Difficult Labours, Premature Birth and Asphyxia Neonatorum on the Mental and Physical Condition of the Child, Especially in Relation to Deformities. *Transactions of the Obstetric Society of London*, **3**, 293. Reprinted in *Cerebral Palsy Bulletin*, **1**, 5–36.

Lonsdale, S. (1978) Family Life with a Handicapped Child. The Parents Speak. *Child Care, Health and Development*, **4**, 99–120.

Lorber, J. (1971) Results of Treatment for Myelomeningocele. *Developmental Medicine and Child Neurology*, **13**, 279–303.

Loring, J. and Burn, G. (1975) *Integration of Handicapped Children in Society*, Routledge & Kegan Paul, London.

Lou, H. C., Lassen, N. A., Tweed, W. A. *et al.* (1979) Pressure Passive Cerebral Blood Flow and Breakdown of the Blood Brain Barrier in Experimental Fetal Asphyxia. *Acta Paediatrica Scand.*, **68**, 35.

Lyen, K. R., Lingam, S., Butterfill, A. M. and Marshall, W. C. (1981) Multicystic Encephalomalacia due to a Foetal Viral Encephalitis. *European Journal of Paediatrics*, **137**, 11–16.

McArdle, G. B., Richardson, C. J., Hayden, C. K. *et al.* (1987) Abnormalities of the Neonatal Brain: MR Imaging. Part II Hypoxic Ischaemic Brain Injury. *Radiology*, **163**, 395–404.

McConkey, R. and McCormack, B. (1983) Breaking Barriers: Educating People about Disability. *Human Horizons Series*, Souvenir, London.

McCormick, B. (1983) Hearing Screening by health Visitors: A Critical Appraisal of the Distraction Test. *Health Visitor*, **56**, 449–51.

MacKeith, R. (1973) The Feelings and Behaviour of Parents of Handicapped Children. *Developmental Medicine and Child Neurology*, **15**, 24–7.

McMichael, J. K. (1971) *Handicap: A Study of Physically Handicapped Children and their Families*, Staples Press, London.

Madge, N. and Fassam, M. (1984) *Physically handicapped children*, Batsford, London.

Marguelec, A. (1966) *Cerebral Palsy in Adolescence and Childhood*. Academic Press, Jerusalem.

Matas, I., Arend, R. A. and Sroufe, L. A. (1978) Continuity of Adaptation in the Second Year. The Relationship between Quality of Attachment and Later

Competence. *Child Development*, **49**, 547–56.

Ment, L. R., Duncan, C. C. and Ehrenkranz, R. A. (1984) Perinatal Cerebral Infarction. *Annals of Neurology*, **16**(5), 559–68.

Minde, K. K. (1978) Coping Styles of 24 Adolescents with Cerebral Palsy. *American Journal of Psychiatry*, **135**, 1344–9.

Minde, K. K., Hacket, J. D., Kilon, D. and Silver, S. (1972) How They Grow Up. Forty-one Physically Handicapped Children and Their Families. *American Journal of Psychiatry*, **128**, 1554–9.

Montessori, M. (1910) *The Advanced Method*. Longmans, Harlow.

Morris, S. E. and Klein, M. D. (1987) Pre-feeding Skills. *Communication Skill Builders*, Tucson, Arizona.

Moxley-Haegert, L. and Serbin, L. A. (1983) Developmental Education for Parents of Delayed Infants: Effects on Parental Motivation and Child Development. *Child Development*, **54**, 1324–31.

Mulcahy, C. M. (1986) An Approach to the Assessment of Sitting Ability for the Prescription of Seating. *British Journal of Occupational Therapy*, **49**, 367–8.

Mulcahy, C. M. and Pountney, T. E. (1986) The Sacral Pad. *Physiotherapy*, **72**(9), 473–4.

Mulcahy, C. M. and Pountney, T. E. (1987) Ramped Cushion. *British Journal of Occupational Therapy*, **50**, 97.

Mulcahy, C. M., Pountney, T. E., Nelham, R. L., Green, M. and Billington, G. D. (1988) Adaptive Seating for the Motor Handicapped. *Physiotherapy*, **74**, 531–6.

Myhr, U. and von Wendt, L. (1991) Improvement of Functional Sitting Position for Children with Cerebral Palsy. *Developmental Medicine and Child Neurology*, **33**, 246–56.

Nelson, K. B. and Ellenberg, J. H. (1981) Apgar Scores as Predictors of Chronic Neurological Disability. *Paediatrics*, **68**(1), 36–44.

Nelson, K. B. and Ellenberg, J. H. (1982) The Children who Outgrew Cerebral Palsy. *Pediatrics*, **69**(5), 529–36.

Nelson, K. B. and Ellenberg, J. H. (1986) Antecedents of Cerebral Palsy. *New England Journal of Medicine*, **315**(2), 81–6.

Neville, B. G. R. (1988) Selective Dorsal Rhizotomy for Spastic Cerebral Palsy. *Developmental Medicine and Child Neurology*, **30**, 395–8.

Newson, J. and Newson E. (1976) *Patterns of Infant Care in an Urban Community*, Penguin, Harmondsworth, Middlesex.

Newton, V. W. (1985) Aetiology of Bilateral Sensorineural Hearing Loss in Young Children. *J. Laryngol. Otol.* (1985 Suppl.), **10**, 40–1.

Nielson, H. (1971) Psychological Appraisal of Children with Cerebral Palsy. *Developmental Medicine and Child Neurology*, **13**, 707–20.

Nolan, C. (1981) *Damburst of Dreams*, Weidenfeld & Nicolson, London.

Norman, M. G. (1980) Bilateral Encephaloclastic Lesions in a 26 Week Gestation Fetus; Effect on Neuronal Migration. *J. Can. Sci. Neurol.*, **7**, 191–4.

Nwaobi, O. M. (1987) Seating Orientations and Upper Extremity Function in Children with Cerebral Palsy. *Physical Therapy*, **67**, 1209–12.

Osofsky, J. D. (1979) *Handbook of Infant Development*, John Wiley, New York.

Oswin, M. (1967) *Behaviour Problems Amongst Children with Cerebral Palsy*. John Wright, Bristol.

Palmer, S., Thompson, R. J. and Linscheid, R. (1975) Applied Behavioural Analysis in the Treatment of Childhood Feeding Problems. *Developmental Medicine and Child Neurology*, **17**, 333–9.

Palmer, F., Shapiro, M., Wachtel, M., Allen, M., Hiller, J., Harryman, M., Mosher, B., Meinert, C. and Capute, M. (1988) The Effects of Physical Therapy on Cerebral Palsy. *New England Journal of Medicine*, **318**(13), 803–8.

Pape, K. E. and Wigglesworth, J. S. (1979) *Haemorrhage, Ischaemia and the Perinatal Brain*, Spastics International Medical Publications, William Heinemann Medical Books, London.

Papousek, H. (1969) Individual Variability in Learned Responses in Human Infants, in *Brain and Early Behaviour* (ed. R. J. Robinson), Academic Press, London.

Peacock, W. J., Arens, L. J. and Berman, B. (1987) Cerebral Palsy Spasticity, Selective Posterior Rhizotomy. *Paediatric Neuroscience*, **13**, 61–6.

Pharoah, P. O. D., Cooke, T., Rosenbloom, L. and Cooke, R. W. I. (1987) Trends in Birth Prevalence of Cerebral Palsy. *Archives of Disease in Childhood*, **62**, 379–84.

Piaget, J. (1953) *The Origin of Intelligence in the Child*, Routledge & Kegan Paul, London.

Piaget, J. (1973) *The Psychology of the Child*, Routledge & Kegan Paul, London.

Piaget, J. and Inhelder, B. (1969) *The Psychology of the Child*, Routledge & Kegan Paul, London.

Pope, P. M. (1985a) A Study of Instability in Relation to Posture in the Wheelchair. *Physiotherapy*, **71**(3), 124–9.

Pope, P. M. (1985b) Proposals for the Improvement of Unstable Postural Condition and Some Cautionary Notes. *Physiotherapy*, **71**(3), 129–31.

Porges, S. W. (1979) Developmental Designs for Infancy Research, in *Handbook of Infant Development* (ed. J. D. Osofsky), John Wiley, New York.

Powell, T. G., Pharoah, P. O. D., Cooke, R. W. I. and Rosenbloom, L. (1988) Cerebral Palsy in Low Birthweight Infants. Spastic Diplegia; Associations with Foetal Immaturity. *Developmental Medicine and Child Neurology*, **30**, 19–25.

Pringle, M. L., Kellmer, and Fiddes, D. O. (1970) The Challenge of Thalidomide. The National Bureau for Cooperation in Childcare, London.

Reynolds, P. C. (1976) Play, Language and Human Evolution, in *Play: Its Role in Development and Evolution* (eds J. S. Bruner, A. Jolly and K. Syva), Penguin, Hardmondsworth, Middlesex.

Reynolds, E. (1987) Early Treatment and Prognosis of Epilepsy. *Epilepsia*, **28**, 97–106.

Richardson, S. A. (1972) People with Cerebral Palsy Talk for Themselves. *Developmental Medicine and Child Neurology*, **14**, 4.

Roberts, J. (1985) *A Celebration of Difference*, Bristol Broadsides (Coop) Ltd.

Robertson, C. and Finer, N. (1985) Term Infants with Hypoxic Ischaemic Encephalopathy. Outcome at 3.5 years. *Developmental Medicine and Child*

Neurology, **27**, 473–84.

Robinson, C. and Fieber, N. (1988) Cognitive Assessment of Motorically Impaired Infants and Preschoolers, in *Assessment of Young Developmentally Disabled Children* (eds T. D. Wachs and R. Sheehan), Plenum Press, New York.

Robinson, M., Smith, M. F. and Cameron, M. D. (1980) Foetal Subdural Haemorrhage Presenting as Hydrocephalus. *B. M. J.,* **281**, 35.

Royal College of Physicians (1986) *Physical Disability in 1986 and Beyond.*

Royal Devon and Exeter Hospital (1985) The Needs of Handicapped Young Adults. *First Report: Paediatric Research Unit,* Department of Child Health, Exeter.

Rutter, M. Graham, P. and Yule, W. (1970) A Neuropsychiatric Study in Childhood. *Clinics in Developmental Medicine No. 35/36,* London Spastics International Medical Publications in association with Heinemann.

Rutter, M. (1985) Resilience in the Face of Adversity. Protective Factors and Resistance to Psychiatric Disorder. *British Journal of Psychiatry,* **147**, 598–611.

Sameroff, A. J. and Chandler, M. (1975) Reproductive Risk and the Continuum of Caregiving Casualty. *Review of Child Development Research,* **4**, 187–244.

Sarnat, H. B. and Sarnat, M. S. (1976) Neonatal Encephalopathy Following Foetal Distress. *Arch. Neurol.,* **33**, 696–705.

Scheers, M. M., Beeker, T. W. and Hertogh, C. M. (1984) Spina Bifida: Feelings, Opinion and Expectations of Parents. *Zeitschrift für Kinderdibrugen, Supplement 39* (December), pp. 120–1.

Schwartz, R. H., Eaton, J., Bower, B. D. and Aynsley-Green, A. (1989) Ketogenic Diets in the Treatment of Epilepsy: Short-Term Clinical Effects. *Developmental Medicine and Child Neurology,* **31**, 145–51.

Segal, S. S. (1971) *From Care to Education,* William Heinemann Medical Books, London.

Seidel, U. P., Chadwick, O. F. and Rutter, M. (1975) Psychological Disorders in Crippled Children. A Comparative Study of Children With and Without Brain Damage. *Developmental Medicine and Child Neurology,* **17**, 563–73.

Shanks, D. E. and Wilson, W. G. (1988) Lobar Holoprosencephaly Presenting as Spastic Diplegia. *Developmental Medicine and Child Neurology,* **30**, 383–6.

Shearer, D. E. and Shearer, M. S. (1976) The Portage Project. A Model for Early Childhood Intervention, in *Intervention Strategies for High Risk Infants and Children* (ed. T. Tjossem), Baltimore University Park Press.

Shentall, G. and Hosking, G. (1986) *British Orthoptic Journal,* **43**, 22–5.

Shepherd, G. M. (1988) *Neurobiology,* Oxford University Press, Oxford.

Sheridan, M. D. (1973) *Developmental Progress from Birth to 5 years,* NFER Nelson, Windsor.

Sheridan, M. D. (1975) *The Developmental Progress of Infants and Young Children.* DHSS No 102.

Slavin, R. E. (1980) Cooperative Learning. *Review of Educational Research,* **50**, 315–42.

Smith, J. F. and Rodeck, C. (1975) Multiple Cystic and Focal Encephalomalacia in Infancy and Childhood with Brainstem Damage. *Journal Neurological Science,* **25**, 377–88.

Spain, B. (1974) Verbal and Performance Ability in Pre-school Children with Spina Bifida. *Developmental Medicine and Child Neurology*, **16**, 773–80.

Stephen, E. and Hawks, S. (1974) Cerebral Palsy and Mental Subnormality, in *Mental Proficiency. The Changing Outlook* (eds A. M. Clarke and A. D. B. Clarke), Methuen, London.

Stanley, F. and Alberman, E. (1984) *The Epidemiology of the Cerebral Palsies.* Spastics International Medical Publications, Blackwell, Oxford.

Stephenson, J. B. P. and King, M. D. (1989) *Handbook of Neurological Investigations in Children.* Wright, Butterworth Scientific Publications, London.

Stern, D. (1977) *The First Relationship. Infant and Mother*, Fontana, London.

Stevens, J. C., Webb, H. D., Smith, M. F. *et al.* (1987) Comparison of Otoacoustic Emissions and Brain Stem Electric Response Audiometry in the Normal Newborn and Babies Admitted to a Special Care Baby Unit. *Clinical Physics and Physiological Measurement*, **8**, 95–104.

Stewart, P. C. and McQuilton, G. (1987) Straddle Seating for the Cerebral Palsied Child. *British Journal of Occupational Therapy*, **50**, 136–8.

Stott, D. H., Moyes, F. A. and Henderson, S. E. (1985) *Diagnosis and Remediation of Handwriting Problems*, Brook Educational, Skelph, Ontario.

Sussova, J., Seibl, Z. and Faber, J. (1990) Hemiparetic Forms of Cerebral Palsy in Relation to Epilepsy and Mental Retardation. *Developmental Medicine and Child Neurology*, **32**, 792–5.

Sylva, K., Bruner, J. S. and Senova, P. (1976) The Role of Play in the Problem Solving of Children 3–5 years old, in *Play: Its Role in Development and Evolution* (eds M. J. Bruner, A. Jolly and K Sylva), Penguin, Harmondsworth, Middlesex.

Temple, F. (1946) Observations on the Rehabilitation of Movement in Cerebral Palsy Problems. *West Virginia Medical Journal*, **42**(4), 77.

Teplin, S. W., Howard, J. A. and O'Connor, M. J. (1981) Self Concept of Young Children with Cerebral Palsy. *Developmental Medicine and Child Neurology*, **23**, 730–8.

Timm, M. A., Strain, P. S. and Eller, P. H. (1979) Effects of Systematic Response Dependant Fading and Thinning Procedures on the Maintenence of Child–Child Interaction. *Journal of Applied Behavioural Analysis*, **12**, 308.

Tirosh, E. and Rabino, S. (1989) Physiotherapy for Children with Cerebral Palsy. *American Journal of Disease in Children*, **143**, 552–5.

Topping, K. J. and Wolfendale, S. (1985) *Parental Involvement in Children's Reading*, Croom Helm, London.

Tripp, J. H. (1985) *Unmet Needs of Handicapped Young Adults.* A report of the European Collective Committee for Child Health of the Children's Research Fund, Liverpool.

Twitchin, D. (1981) *Making the Grade.* King's Fund Report KFC/82/13.

Uzgiris, I. C. (1981) Two Functions of Imitation During Infancy. *International Journal of Behavioural Development*, **4**(1), 1–12.

Uzgiris, I. C. and Hunt, J. M. (1975) *Assessment in Infancy: Ordinal Scale of Psychological Development*, University of Illinois Press.

Veelken, N., Hagberg, B., Hagberg, G. and Olow, I. (1983) Diplegic Cerebral Palsy in Swedish Term and Preterm Children. *Neuropediatrics*, **14**, 20–8.

Volpe, J. J. (1981) *Neurology of the Newborn*, W. B. Saunders Co. Philadelphia, pp. 195–8.

Volpe, J. J., Herscovitch, P., Perlman, J. M. and Raickle, M. E. (1983) Positron Emission Tomography in the Newborn. *Paediatrics*, **72**, 589–601.

Waisbren, S. E. (1980) Parent Teachers After the Birth of a Developmentally Disabled Child. *American Journal of Mental Deficiency*, **84**, 345–51.

Warner, J. (1981) *Helping the Handicapped Child with Early Feeding*. Winslow Press, London.

Wasserman, S. A., Allen, R. and Solomon, C. R. (1985) At Risk Toddlers and Their Mothers. The Special Case of Physical Handicap. *Child Development*, **56**, 73–83.

Wedell, K. (1973) *Learning and Perceptuo-motor Disabilities in Children*, Wiley, London.

Wikler, I., Wasow, M. and Hatfield, E. (1981) Chronic Sorrow Revisited. Parent versus Professional Depiction of the Adjustment of Mentally Retarded Children. *American Journal of Mental Deficiency*, **51**, 63–70.

Wilder, R. M. (1921) The Effects of Ketonemia on the Course of Epilepsy. *Mayo Clinic Bulletin*, **2**, 307–14.

Wolman, B. B. (1982) *Handbook of Developmental Psychology*. Prentice Hall, Englewood Cliffs.

Wright, J. (1982) An Integrative Model of Parental Involvement, in *Building an Alliance for Children* (ed. M. Peters), University of Washington Program Development Scheme, Seattle.

Wright, J. S., Granger, R. D. and Sameroff, A. J. (1984) Parental Acceptance and Developmental Handicap, in *Severely Handicapped Young Children and their Families* (ed. J. Blatcher), Academic Press, London.

Wyatt, J. S., Edwards, A. D., Azzopardi, D. and Reynolds, E. O. R. (1989) Magnetic Resonance and Near Infrared Spectroscopy for Investigation of Perinatal Hypoxic Ischaemic Brain Injury. *Archives of Disease in Childhood*, **64**, 953–63.

Yule, W. and Rutter, M. (1970) Educational Aspects of Physical Disorders, in *Education Health and Behaviour* (eds M. Rutter, J. Tizard and K. Whitmore), Longmans, London.

Zelazo, P. R. (1982) An Information Approach to Infant Cognitive Assessment, in (eds M. Lewis and L. T. Taft), *Developmental Disabilities; Theory, Assessment and Intervention*, MTP Press, Lancaster.

Zelazo, P.R. (1979) Reactivity to Perceptual Cognitive Events; Application for Infant Assessment, in *Infants at Risk. Assessment of Cognitive Functioning* (eds R. B. Kearsley and I. E. Sigel). Erlbaum, New Jersey.

Index